ON A ROLL

Exercising with a Foam Roller

Lisa M. Wolfe

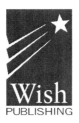

Wish Publishing
Terre Haute, Indiana
www.wishpublishing.com

LCCN: 2006933455

Printed in the United States of America
10 9 8 7 6 5 4 3 2 1

Published by
Wish Publishing
P.O. Box 10337
Terre Haute, IN 47801, USA
www.wishpublishing.com

Distributed in the United States by
Cardinal Publishers Group
222 Hillside Avenue, Suite 100
Indianapolis, IN 46218
www.cardinalpub.com

To Morgan and Dylan for their understanding and love.

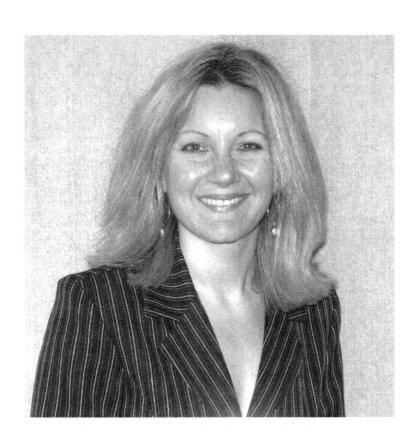

Introduction

I remember my first experience with a foam roller. I was in physical therapy following a knee surgery. My therapist brought out what looked like a large Styrofoam pool noodle. I wondered what she could possibly want me to do with it.

My doubts were quickly replaced with admiration for this clever prop. My quadriceps and hamstrings felt more awake while using the foam roller than they had during any pre-surgery exercise. Another benefit was the reduction in discomfort.

I was hooked. I began roller training all the muscles of my body, and I also introduced all my clients and my class participants to foam rollers. They quickly learned that this new "toy" was now a part of our weekly exercise routines. The strength, balance and flexibility gains by adding rollers to a workout were visible to my participants and me.

Whether you're seeking an entirely new workout or a variation on your old standard, I hope this roller workout finds you intrigued and ready to rock and roll.

In health,
Lisa M. Wolfe

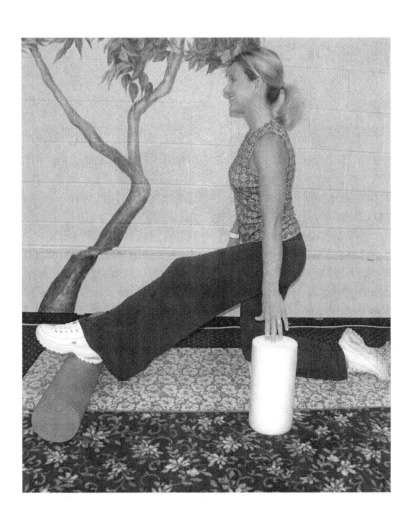

ROLLER TRAINING

What is roller training?

Training on foam rollers is like balancing on logs. The unstable surface provides a unique tool for balance, stability, core, strength, flexibility and body position awareness exercises. If your joints are not aligned and your body position is not perfect when using a roller, you will fall.

Use of the roller awakens the unity of the mind and body. As opposed to passive muscle strengthening where the body goes through the motions of an exercise without conscious thought, active muscle strengthening uses the focus of the mind in order to increase the challenge to the body. In order to maintain the body's balance on a changeable surface, the central nervous system is activated.

A roller provides a diversion for strength training. The roller alone can be used as the strengthening device, or it can be used as a bench for traditional strengthening exercises. One can stand, kneel, sit or lie on a roller for additional core strength in an exercise routine. Roller exercises use the core in every movement to encourage a healthy back and strong stomach.

The addition of a roller can really enhance a flexibility program. One will be able to sink deeper into stretches when a roller is properly placed under the body.

Yoga and Pilates exercises will also benefit from a roller. The varying surface of a roller will intensify the exercises as well as increase joint position awareness, which is crucial for proper form and alignment in yoga and Pilates. The rollers engage the core in every movement to build strength. This will lead to more advanced poses. Another benefit is heightened flexibility because the rollers allow the body to maneuver into positions that otherwise would not be possible.

While there are many benefits to roller exercises, it must be understood that they are not cardiovascular exercises.

What are foam rollers?

Foam rollers resemble the noodles that people use while floating in water. Fitness rollers are thicker, with a usual diameter of six inches, but a roller's diameter can vary between four to seven inches. The diameter can also be changed when the roller is cut in half to provide a more stable base for a beginner. The length can vary from 12 to 36 inches to allow for a variety of exercises.

Foam rollers can also vary in density. The higher a roller's density, the longer the roller will maintain its shape. Over time, the weight on the roller causes the foam to break down. This results in indents from feet and hands. Manufacturers are increasing the density of rollers so they maintain their shape for a longer period of time.

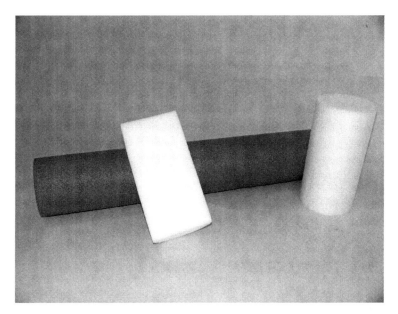

These are three different types of rollers. The one in the background is a full three-foot roller. The one on the left is a one-foot roller, cut in half lengthwise; on the right is a full one-foot roller.

Do other types of rollers exist?

Rollers can also be made out of polyurethane or burst-resistant vinyl (for an inflatable roller). The polyurethane provides a nonslip surface. An inflatable roller can be adjusted for individual comfort. The more firm the roller, the more challenging the exercises.

Who can use a roller?

The rollers can be used by everyone, from beginners to advanced participants. A beginner cuts the rollers in half and places the flat side down for a more stable base. The intermediate user turns the flat side up to provide a stable base for the feet. The advanced user performs the exercises on a full roller.

Certain people with pre-existing conditions should not use rollers. These will be addressed in Chapter Nine.

Are there other benefits?

The rollers are lightweight, which makes them easy for all to use. There is no setup required, so the workout time is spent on exercise.

Rollers are inexpensive and are easily cleaned with soap and water, especially the vinyl rollers. They are effortlessly transported and can be used at home or in a health club. After a workout, they can be efficiently stored either upright or lying flat.

An added benefit is that the rollers can be used for a complete body massage. When the rollers are moved up and down the body, the muscles respond with lengthening and relaxation.

What should I know before a workout?

The roller should be used in an area free of clutter. Since the rollers carry a risk of falling, the workout area should be large enough to move around freely without the fear of falling into anything or anyone. Shoes and clothes should always be worn when exercising with a roller. Keep a towel nearby to wipe down the roller should it become slippery.

When executing the exercises, always begin with a large muscle group such as the chest, back or legs and progress to a small muscle group such as the shoulders, calves or arms. Perform 2-3 sets of 6-10 repetitions of each exercise unless otherwise noted. For the first few workouts, perform two sets of six repetitions. Once those are comfortable and can be completed smoothly, progress to additional repetitions and then finally to an additional set.

Use the strengthening program 3-4 days a week, allowing for a day of rest between workouts. The flexibility and massage training can be performed every day.

Over time, change from a full roller to a half roller and back again in order to provide variety.

Always keep the spine straight and the stomach pulled in tight. Remember to breathe and exhale during the hardest part of the movement.

Now you're ready to get started!

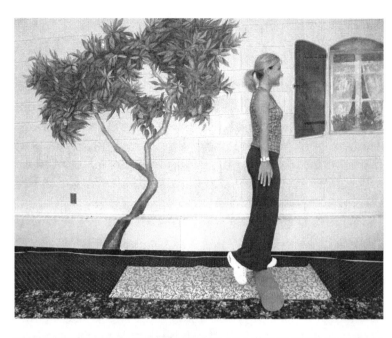

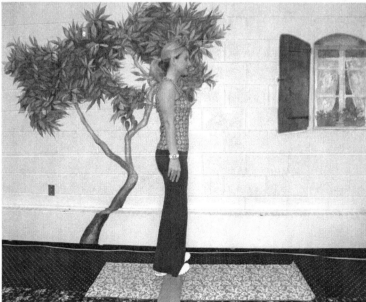

WARM-UP AND BALANCE TRAINING

2

Why warm up?

We begin by using large body movements to increase the temperature of the muscles and to heighten the blood flow to the muscles, connective tissue and extremities. This will help prevent muscle tears or pulls. These large body movements also lubricate the joints for ease of movement.

Perform two sets of 10 repetitions of the exercises on pages 14-19.

TIPS FROM LISA:

- Move every joint in the body through a full range of motion before participating in the more intense movements.
- If exercising first thing in the morning, walk through the house or travel up and down the stairs to prepare the muscles and joints for the workout.

Arm Reaches

Lying on your back with the roller placed vertically against the spine, bend your knees and place your feet flat on the floor. Extend both arms over your head to touch the floor. One arm at a time, raise the arm toward the ceiling until the hand is directly over the shoulder. Return your arm to the starting position and repeat with the opposite arm.

TIPS FROM LISA:

- Widen the distance between the knees for increased stability.
- Look directly at the ceiling to keep the neck in alignment.

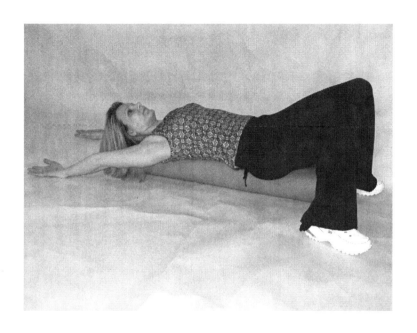

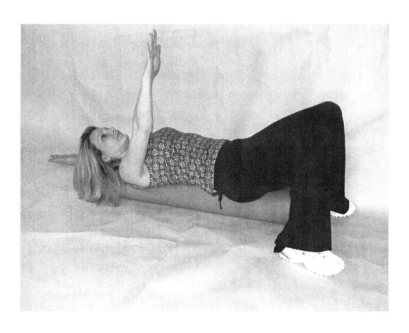

Leg Reaches

Lying on your back with the roller placed vertically against the spine, extend your arms overhead and straighten your legs. One leg at a time, raise the leg toward the ceiling until the foot is directly over the hip. Return your leg to the starting position and repeat with the opposite leg.

TIPS FROM LISA:

- Use the breath to control the speed of movement. Inhale and lift the leg. Exhale and lower.
- Center the weight of the supporting leg into the heel for increased stability.

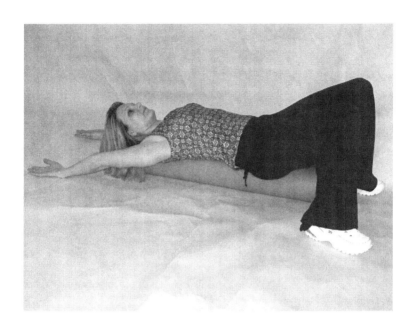

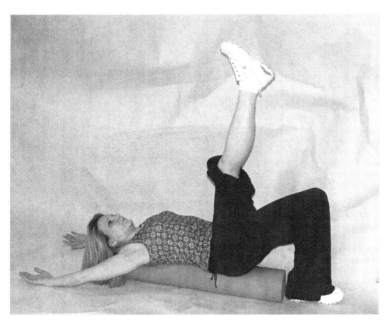

Snow Angels

Lying on your back with the roller placed vertically against the spine, extend your arms overhead and straighten your legs. Extend your legs to the sides as you lower your arms toward your sides, keeping the backs of your hands toward the floor. This resembles making an angel in the snow.

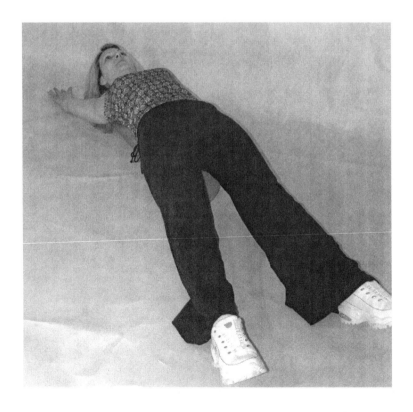

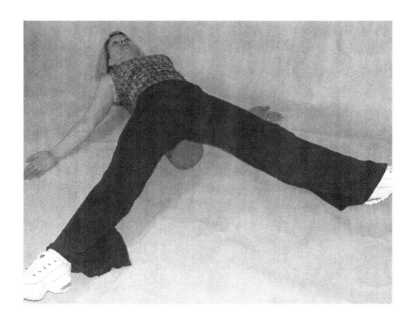

TIPS FROM LISA:

- Point the toes to activate the muscles in the legs.
- Tighten the abdominal muscles to aid with balance.

What about balance?

Balance is being able to maintain the body's center of gravity. Each time the body shifts position and moves out of balance, muscles are activated to bring the body back into balance. The roller adds an unstable surface, so the balance system is further challenged to maintain equilibrium. The importance of a strong sense of balance is to reduce the risk of falling. The following balance training exercises can also be used to warm the body.

Log Roll

Place the roller horizontally on the floor. Step both feet onto the roller. Slowly begin walking in small steps forward across the room. For an added challenge, walk backward across the room returning to the start position.

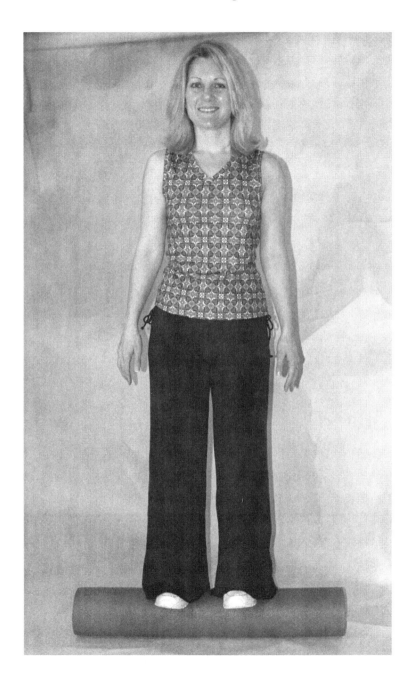

Standing

Place the roller horizontally on the floor. Step both feet onto the roller. Maintain balance while extending both arms overhead. Hold for a count of 10-15. For an added challenge, balance on one foot at a time.

TIPS FROM LISA:

- Maintain proper breathing using a complete inhale and exhale.
- Reach up through the fingertips to lengthen the spine.

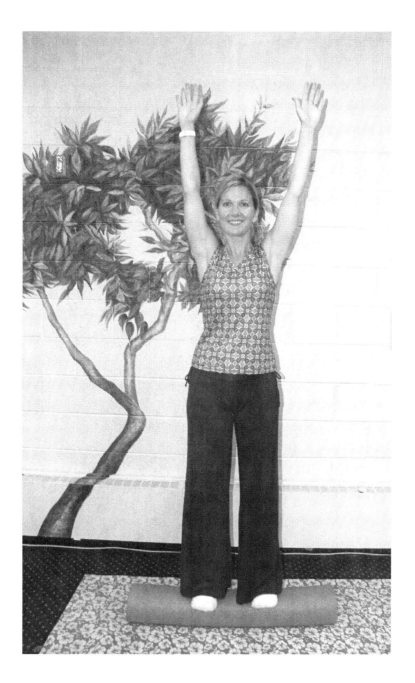

Around the World

Place the roller horizontally on the floor. Step both feet onto the roller. Shift your weight onto your left leg. Keep your back straight, your stomach tight and look forward. Extend your straight right leg in front of the body, to the right side and then straight out behind. Set the right foot on the roller and repeat the sequence on the left. Repeat for 10 repetitions on both sides.

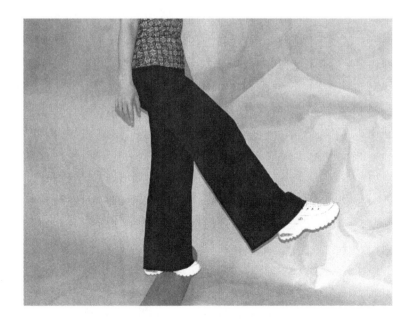

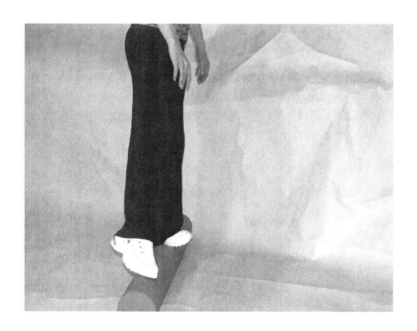

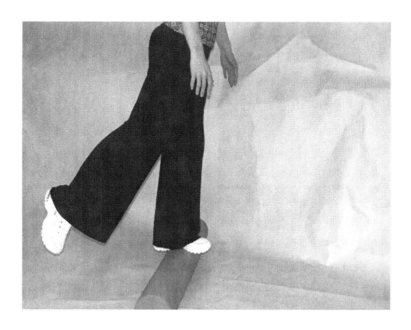

Kneeling

Place the roller horizontally on the floor. Kneel on top of the roller, placing it slightly below the knees. Maintain balance while extending both arms overhead. Hold for a count of 10-15.

TIPS FROM LISA:

- Perform the exercise in a clear room.
- Contract the backs of the legs to lift the feet off the floor.

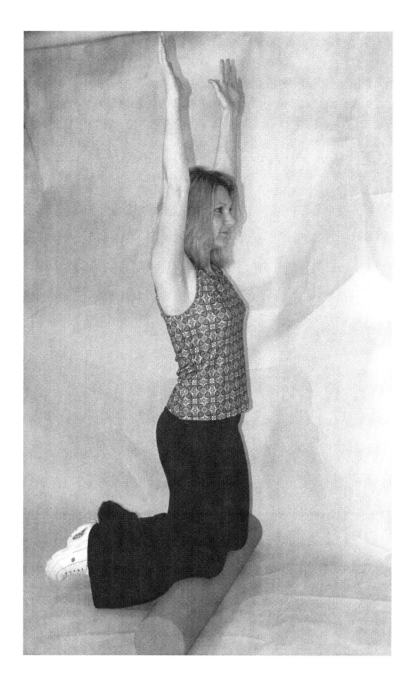

Half-Roller Kneeling

Place a half roller vertically on the floor with the flat side facing up. Kneel on the roller. Shift the weight of the body from side to side and use the arms to maintain balance.

TIPS FROM LISA:

- Contract the abdominal muscles to help with stability.
- Raise the arms to the side to maintain balance.

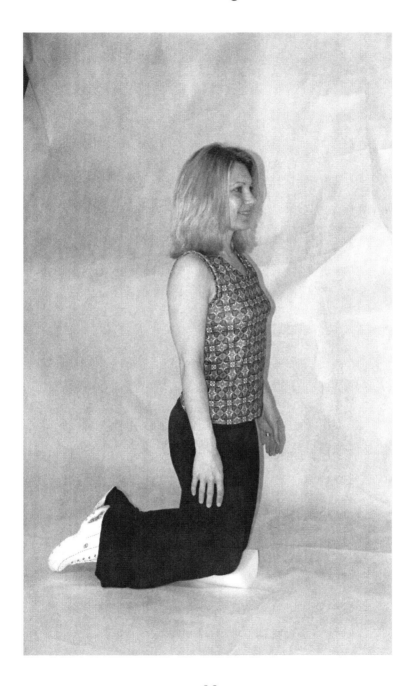

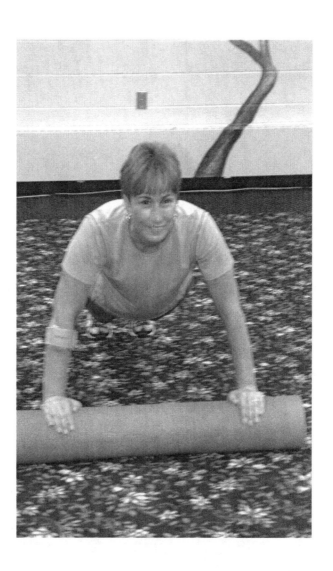

UPPER BODY
STRENGTHENING

3

How are rollers used to strengthen the muscles of the upper body?

Using a roller for strength training adds diversity to a workout. Traditional exercises performed on a roller increase the challenge which causes the muscles to respond with improved strength and tone. The roller can be used in place of a bench or ball for standing, sitting, kneeling or lying exercises with dumbbells or resistance bands.

Used on its own, the roller provides a unique training tool. When exercises are performed using the weight of the body along with the various positions of a roller, the muscles of the upper body are strengthened.

Perform 2-3 sets of 6-10 repetitions.

Neck Extension

Lying on your stomach with the roller placed vertically against the body, position your chin so that it is at the end of the roller. Place your forearms on the floor to stabilize your body. Inhaling, tuck your chin and lower your forehead toward the floor. Relax the neck. Exhaling, squeeze your shoulder blades together and lift your head until your neck is in line with your spine. Do not attempt to look up toward the ceiling.

TIPS FROM LISA:
- Close the eyes to improve focus.
- Inhale as the head lifts and exhale when it lowers.

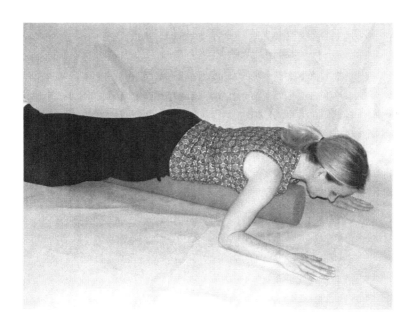

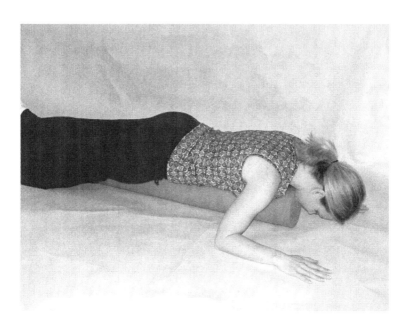

"V" Push-ups

Place the roller horizontally on the floor. Position your hands on the roller shoulder-distance apart. Place your feet approximately 2-3 feet behind the hands. Straighten your legs so that your hips are raised toward the ceiling. Allow the top of your head to drop toward the ground and relax the neck. As you inhale, bend the elbows, lowering the shoulders toward the hands. As you exhale, straighten the arms and return to start.

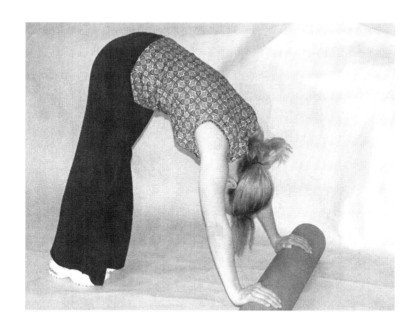

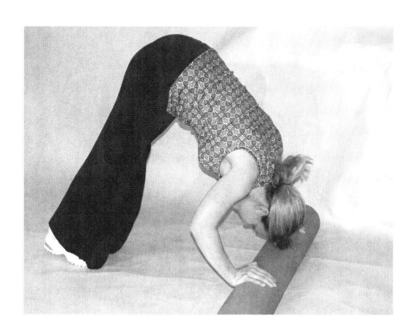

Traditional Shoulder Press

Kneeling on a horizontally placed roller, hold a dumbbell in each hand. Begin with the hands near the shoulders. Keeping the palms facing forward, exhale and raise the arms overhead. Inhale and return to start.

TIPS FROM LISA:
- Place the roller below the knee joint.
- For an added challenge, lift one foot.

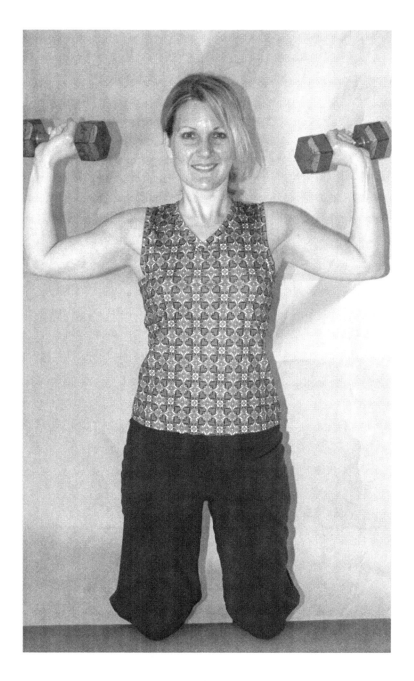

Push-ups

Place the roller horizontally on the floor. Place your hands on the roller shoulder-distance apart. Straighten your legs behind you and press your toes into the floor. As you inhale, bend the elbows, lowering the chest toward the floor. As you exhale, straighten the arms and return to start. For beginners, place the knees on the floor. For a variation, place your hands on the floor and your feet on the roller. Remember to contract the stomach muscles to aid in balance.

TIPS FROM LISA:

- Keep eyes focused on the floor to protect the neck.
- Press the hips toward the floor.

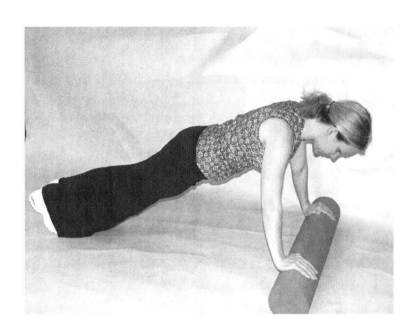

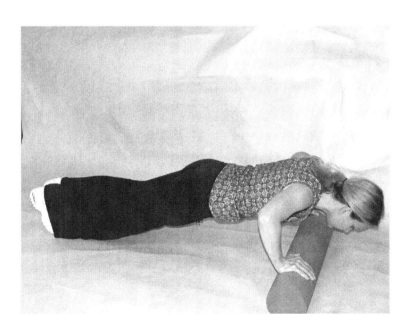

Traditional Chest Flys

Lie on your back on a vertically placed roller. Hold a dumbbell in each hand and place your feet on the floor. Begin with your arms straight over the chest. As you inhale, lower your arms to the floor. Keep your arms straight as you lower them. As you exhale, return your arms over your chest.

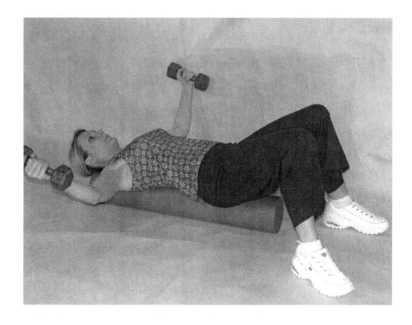

Traditional Tricep Kickback

Lie face down on a vertically placed roller. Straighten your legs and press your toes into the floor. Hold a dumbbell in each hand. Begin with the elbows bent and the hands near the armpits. Exhale and straighten the arms, lifting the dumbbells higher than the body. Inhale and return to the start position.

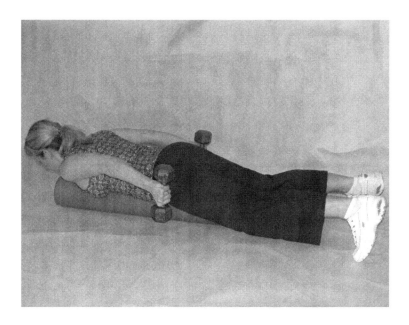

Dips

Place the roller horizontally on the floor. Sit on the roller with your hands positioned next to your hips and resting on the roller and your fingers pointing down toward the floor. Walk your feet away from the roller. Beginners should keep their feet closer to the roller while those more advanced should straighten their legs. As you inhale, bend the elbows and lower the hips toward the floor. As you exhale, straighten the arms and return to the start position. Aim the elbows straight behind the body, not out to the sides (see bottom photo on the next page). For a variation, place your hands on the floor and your feet on the roller.

TIPS FROM LISA:
- Center your weight back into the heels, not forward into the toes.
- Move the entire body as one unit, instead of only moving the hips.

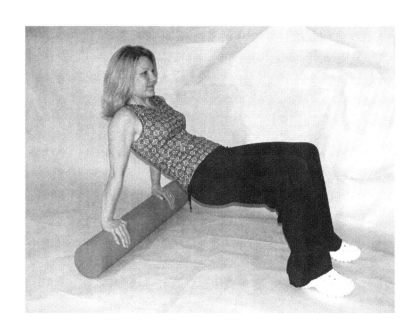

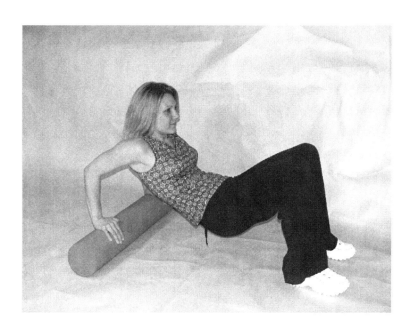

Wall Roll

Place the roller horizontally against a wall at hip height. Place your hands shoulder-distance apart on the underside of the roller. Exhale and press your hands into the roller while rolling it up the wall to near shoulder height. Inhale and roll the roller down the wall to hip height. Keep your knees slightly bent when standing.

TIPS FROM LISA:

- The more pressure put into the roller, the more challenging is the exercise.
- Contract the abdominal muscles to support the back.

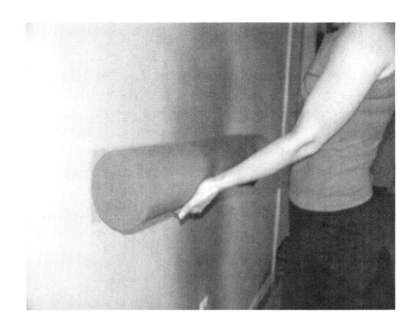

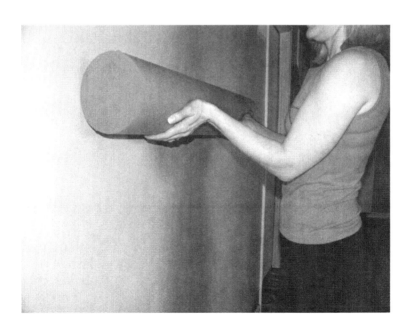

Hyperextension

Place the roller horizontally on the floor. Lie face down on top of the roller with it placed directly above the hips. Widen your legs behind you into the shape of the letter "V" and press the toes into the floor. Cross your arms over your chest and rest your arms on the floor. As you exhale, use the muscles in your back to raise your chest and arms off the floor. Inhale and slowly lower your chest to the start position.

TIPS FROM LISA:

- Keep the focus down toward the floor.
- Lengthen the spine as the body lifts.

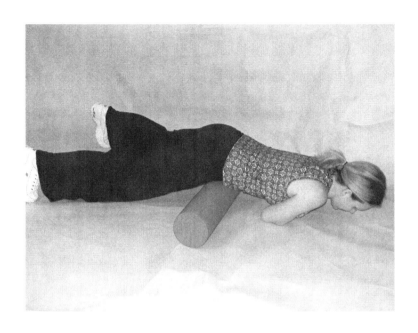

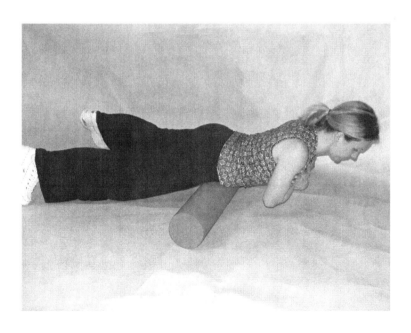

Traditional Bicep Curl

Stand on a horizontally placed roller. Hold a dumb-bell in each hand. Begin with the arms straight at the sides and your palms facing up. Exhale and raise your palms to your shoulders. Inhale and lower your palms to the start position.

TIPS FROM LISA:
- Focus on a distant spot to aid with balance.
- Hold the dumbbells tightly, but not in a restrictive manner.

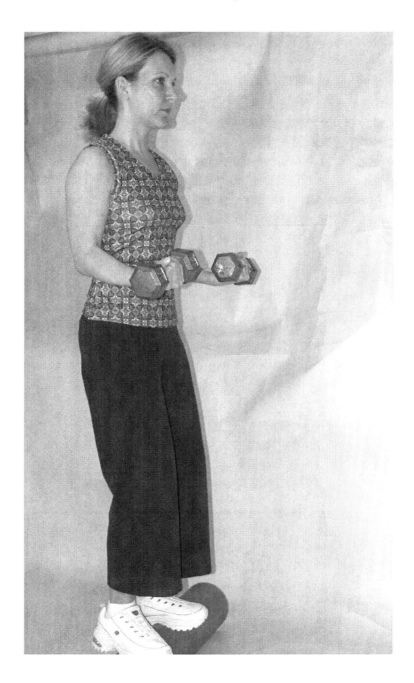

Plank with Arm Raise

Place the roller horizontally on the floor. Position your hands on the roller approximately shoulder-distance apart. Straighten your legs behind you and press your toes into the floor. Maintain your stability by tightening your stomach and looking straight down at the floor. As you exhale, lift your right hand off the roller and away from the body. As you inhale, return your hand to the start position. Repeat on the left arm.

TIPS FROM LISA:

- Shift the weight of the body into the opposite hand before lifting the other.
- Reach away from the body through your fingers and toes.

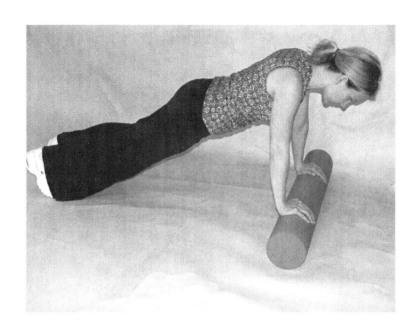

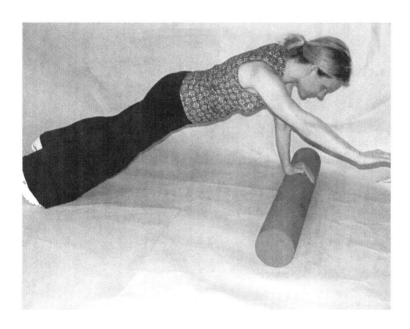

Traditional Lat Pull-in

Step one foot onto a horizontally placed roller. Hold a dumbbell in the opposite hand. Place your other hand above the knee of the supporting leg. Place the opposite foot approximately 2-3 feet behind the body. Begin with the dumbbell next to the knee on the roller. Exhale and bring the dumbbell into your hip. Keep your elbow close to the body. Inhale and return to the start position.

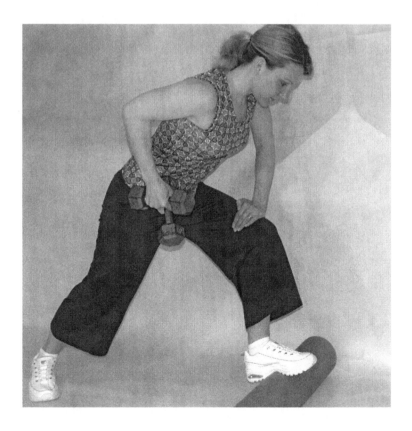

LOWER BODY
STRENGTHENING

How can the roller be an effective lower body strengthening tool?

The roller is an unstable surface, so any exercises performed on it require the use of even the smallest stabilizing muscles. As opposed to traditional lower body exercises which usually target the large muscle groups, the roller exercises require all the muscles of the lower body to work together. In order to remain upright when standing on the roller, the muscles, ligaments, tendons and joints are all active to keep you from falling.

Exercising with the roller requires more conscious involvement than traditional machine-driven leg exercises. For example, when sitting in a leg extension machine, your mind could be on a beach in Hawaii, yet your legs will still perform the exercise. That is not true with the roller exercises. If your mind wanders away from concentrating on body position, balance is lost.

Perform 2-3 sets of 6-10 repetitions.

Squats

Place the roller horizontally on the floor. Place your feet hip-distance apart on the roller. Find a stable focal point on which to concentrate. Keeping your spine straight, inhale and bend your knees, lowering your hips toward the floor. Bend to a comfortable level, but do not go lower than your thighs parallel to the floor. Exhale and straighten the legs to the starting position. Your arms can be at your sides or held out for balance.

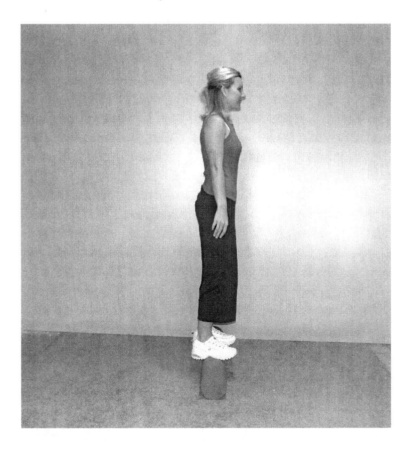

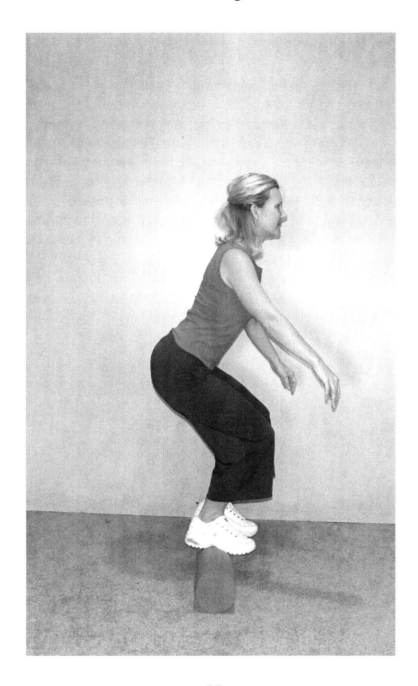

Wall Squats

Place the roller horizontally against a wall. Stand with your back toward the roller at hip height. Rest your back onto the roller and place your feet approximately two feet away from the wall. As you inhale, bend your knees, lower your hips toward the floor and roll the roller toward your shoulder blades. As you exhale, straighten the legs and return to the start position. For a variation, widen your legs and point your knees and toes out to the sides. Your arms can be at your sides or held out for balance.

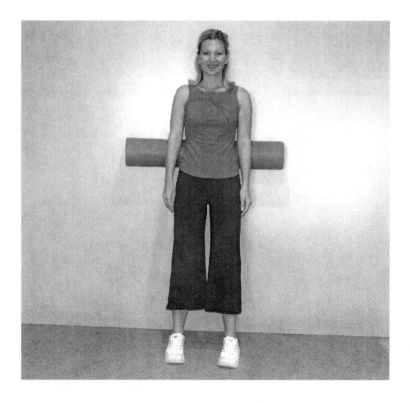

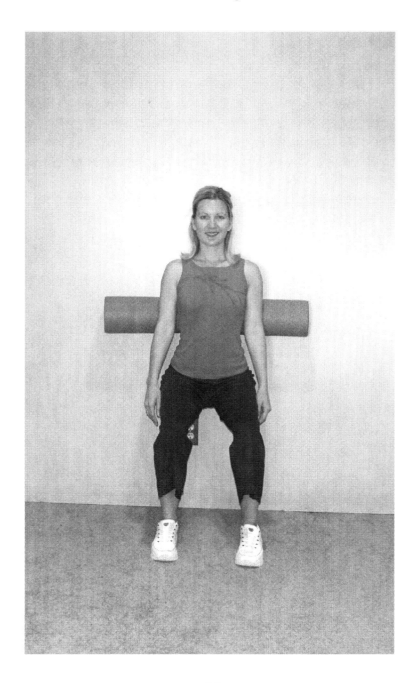

Lunge

Place the roller horizontally on the floor. Step your right foot onto the roller. Place your left foot behind the body into a lunge position and press your toes into the floor. As you inhale, bend your right knee and lower your left leg toward the floor. As you exhale, straighten your right knee and return to the start position. Complete the repetitions then switch to the left leg. Your arms can be at your sides or held out for balance.

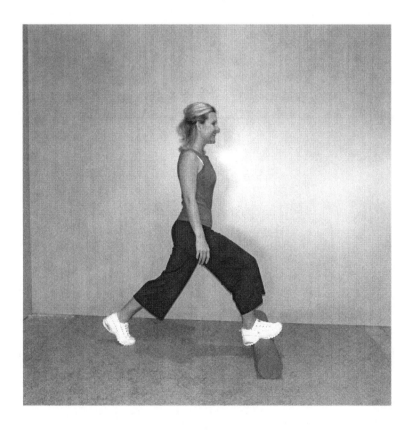

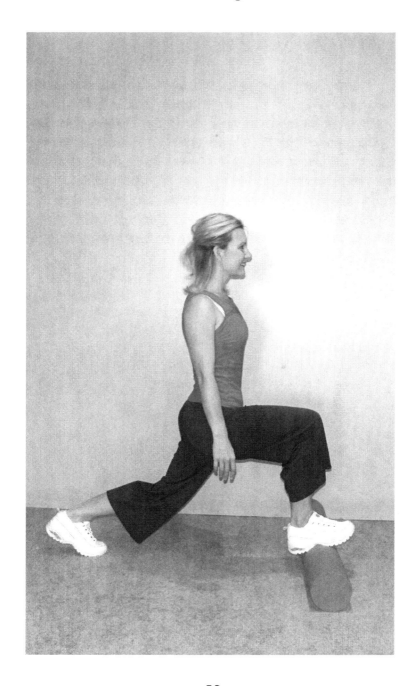

Kneeling Roll

Place a half roller horizontally on the floor. Place a full roller in front of it horizontally on the floor. Kneel on the half roller with your right leg. Extend your left leg in front of the body and place your left heel on the roller. As you exhale, bend your left knee and allow the roller to roll and bring your left foot close to the body. As you inhale, straighten the left knee and return to the start position. Complete the repetitions then switch to the right leg. A chair or third roller can be used to support the hands.

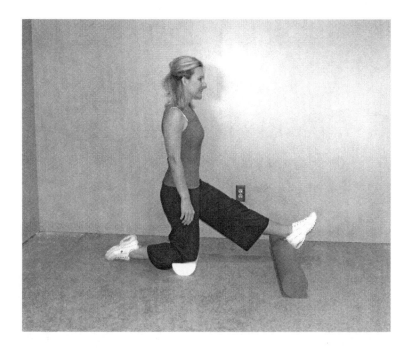

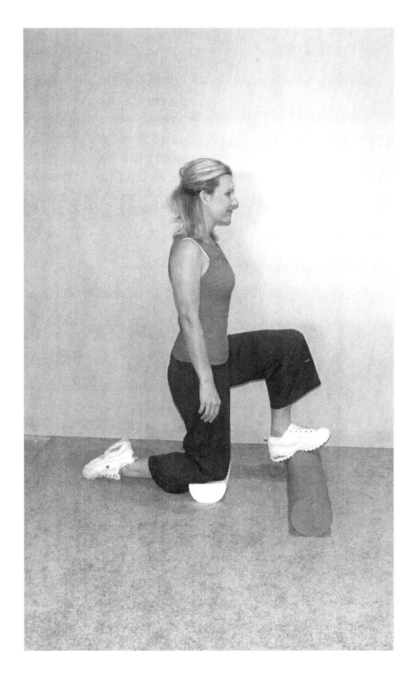

Single Leg Dead Lift

Place a roller horizontally on the floor. Step both feet onto the roller. Shifting the weight onto your right foot, bend your left knee and extend your left foot behind the body. As you inhale, fold forward from the waist and reach toward your right foot with your right hand. As you exhale, use the muscles in the back of your right leg and return the upper body to the start position. Complete the repetitions then switch to the left leg.

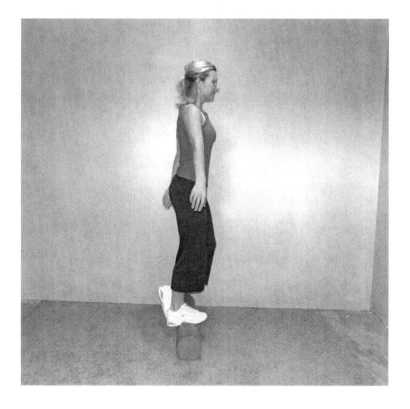

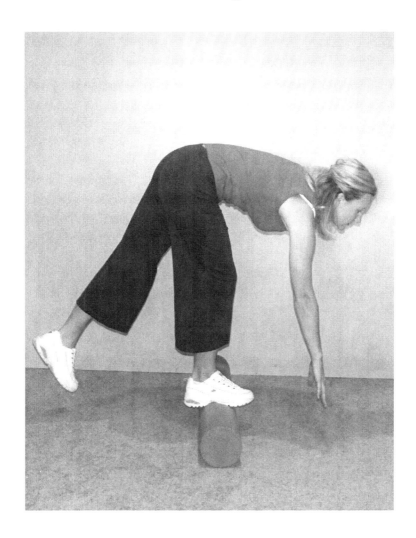

Bridge

Place a roller horizontally on the floor. Lie on your back with your feet on the roller. Position your feet hip-distance apart and align your knees and toes. The roller should be approximately two feet from your torso. Place your arms at your sides. Keeping your neck very still, inhale and raise your hips toward the ceiling. Hold for a count of 20, or lift and lower your hips for repetitions, exhaling on the lowering. For a variation, roll the feet away from and toward the body in the lifted position.

TIPS FROM LISA:

- Press shoulders into the floor for support.
- Lift the hips to a comfortable height and contract the backside of the body.

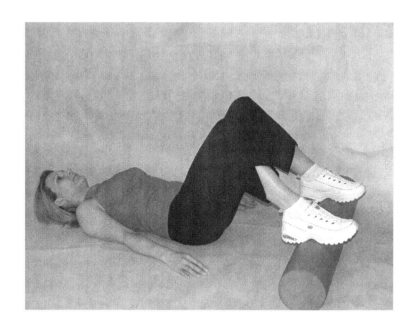

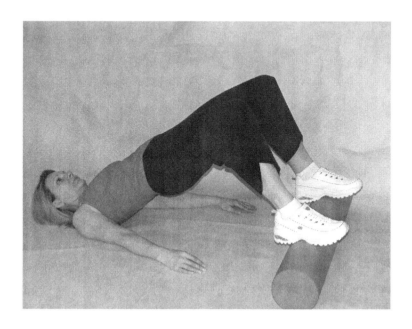

Calf Raise

Place a roller horizontally on the floor. Step both feet onto the roller. Hold onto a chair or a wall for balance, if needed. As you inhale, slowly lower your heels toward the floor, keeping the roller still. As you exhale, lift your heels and come up slightly onto the toes.

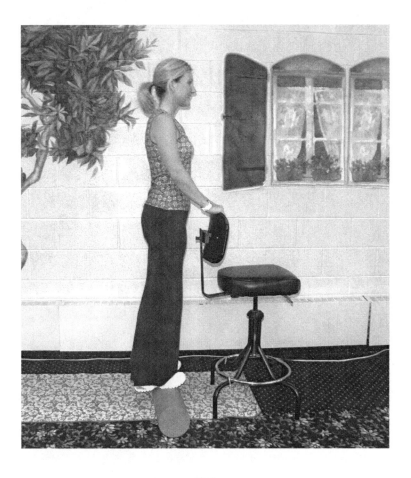

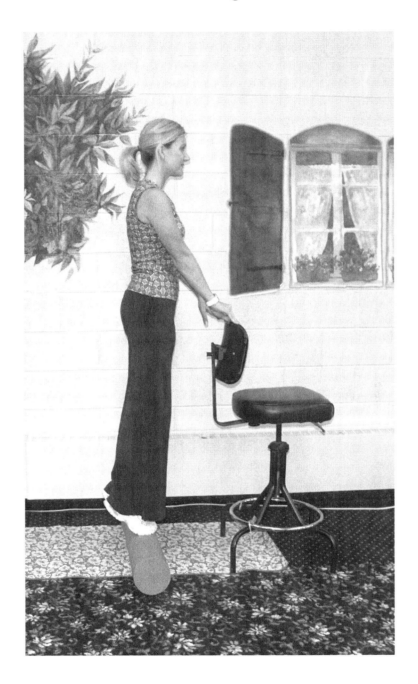

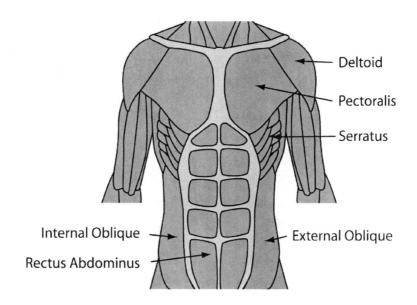

Deltoid

Pectoralis

Serratus

Internal Oblique

External Oblique

Rectus Abdominus

CORE STRENGTH

What is the core?

The core of the body consists of all of the muscles of the stomach and lower back. It also includes the muscles along the spine and the hips. These muscles work together to maintain a strong trunk and provide a stable base from which movement may occur. The core allows for the transfer of power from the lower body to the upper body and back again.

There are no bones in the abdominal area. This cavity is supported only by the muscles that cover it, so strong abdominal muscles are a must. Strong abdominal muscles also give the appearance of a smaller midsection.

What muscles are in the stomach?

The abdominal muscles are a group of four different muscles. One muscle lies up the center of the stomach. Another muscle lies around the stomach holding it in place and supporting posture. The other two cross over each other along the sides, similar to putting our hands in our front and back pockets. It is important to keep these muscles strong in order to prevent strain on the back. Perform 2-3 sets of 8-12 repetitions of the exercises on pages 70-79.

Crunches

Place the roller vertically on the floor. Sit straddling the center of it. Bend your knees and rest your back on the roller. Place your hands behind your head. Keep your chin off your chest and your elbows open wide. As you exhale, tighten your stomach and lift your upper back off the roller. As you inhale, release the back to the start position.

TIPS FROM LISA:
- Find a focal point on the ceiling to keep the neck aligned.
- Widen the distance between the knees to aid balance.

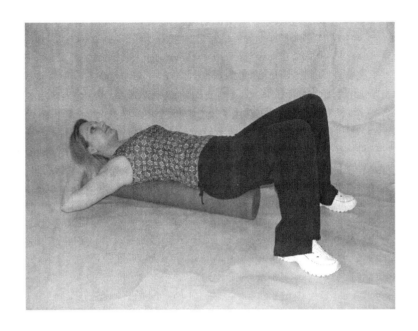

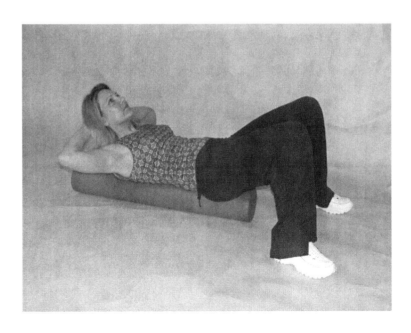

Ab Roll

Place the roller horizontally on the floor. Kneel in front of the roller, with the roller touching your knees. Keeping your hands in a prayer position, place your fingertips onto the roller with your little fingers facing toward the floor. As you inhale, lower your upper body toward the floor as you roll out, until your elbows are on top of the roller. As you exhale, tighten your stomach and roll back to the starting position.

TIPS FROM LISA:

- Look down toward the floor to protect the neck.
- Keep the top of the feet pressed into the floor.

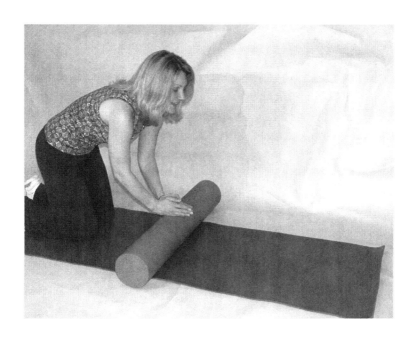

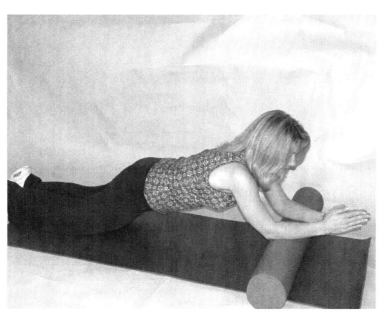

Jack Knife

Place the roller horizontally on the floor. Begin on your hands and knees with the roller next to your feet. Straighten your legs and place the tops of your feet on the roller. As you exhale, raise your hips toward the ceiling and roll your feet closer to the body. As you inhale, lower your hips and return your feet to the start position.

TIPS FROM LISA:

- Tighten the abdominal muscles to keep the spine straight.
- Look down between the hands to protect the neck.

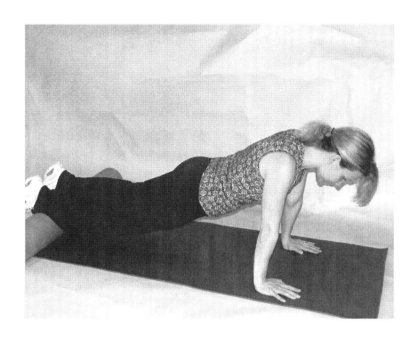

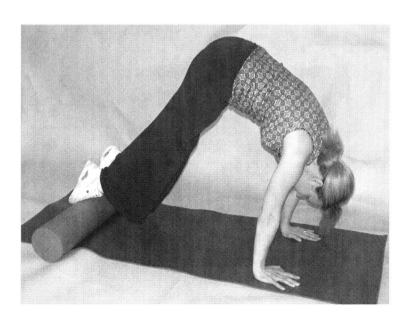

Boat

Place the roller vertically on the floor. Sit straddling the roller with one foot on each side. Hold your arms out to your sides. As you exhale, tighten your stomach and lift both feet off floor. You may keep your legs bent or straighten them. Maintain this position for a count of 20.

TIPS FROM LISA:

- Beginners should place the feet on a roller for support.
- Maintain breathing while keeping the abdominals contracted.

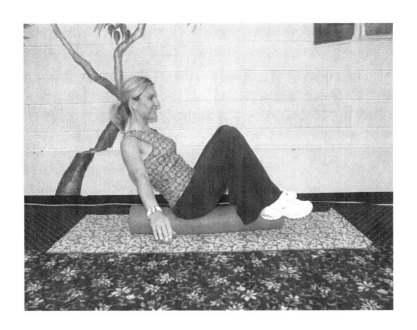

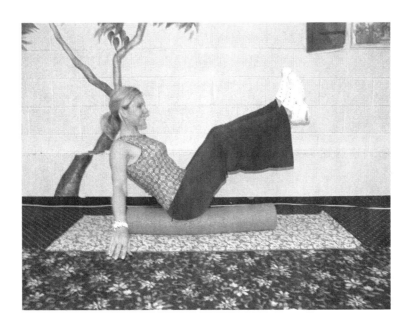

What muscles are in the back?

The muscles in the back that are included in the core primarily run along the spinal column. These muscles allow us to bend and extend the spine and are responsible for good posture.

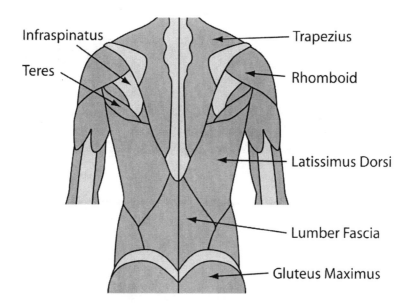

Infraspinatus — Trapezius

Teres — Rhomboid

— Latissimus Dorsi

— Lumber Fascia

— Gluteus Maximus

The Swim

Place the roller horizontally on the floor. Lie on top of the roller, placing it directly above the hips. Straighten your arms and legs. Inhale and lift your arms and legs off the floor. Exhale and quickly raise and lower your arms and legs as if swimming. Continue for a count of 20 and repeat if needed.

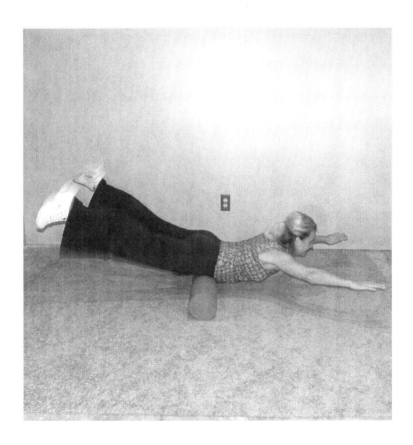

The Cobra

Place the roller horizontally on the floor. Lie on top of the roller, placing it directly above your hips. Straighten your legs and press your toes into the floor. Place your elbows directly underneath your shoulders with your fingers pointing away from the body. Inhale and press through the hands to lift your chest off the floor. Keep the elbows slightly bent. Hold for a count of 20 and repeat if needed.

TIPS FROM LISA:

- Lengthen the spine and lift up from the lower back.
- Center the weight in the palms, not the fingertips.

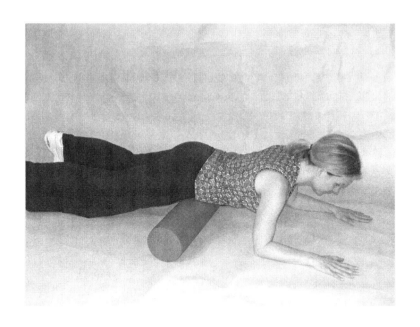

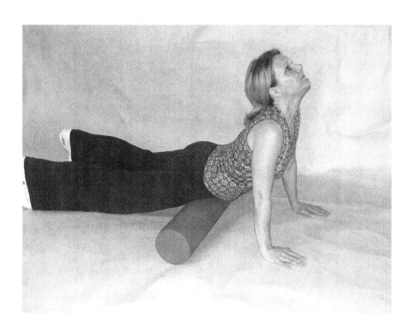

Leg Lifts

Place the roller horizontally on the floor. Lie on top of the roller with it placed directly above the hips. Straighten your legs and press your toes into the floor. Place your elbows underneath your shoulders and your forearms on the floor. Exhale and lift the right leg to a comfortable height. Inhale and release the right leg to the start position. Repeat on the left leg then complete 8-12 repetitions.

TIPS FROM LISA:

- Look down between the hands to protect the neck.
- Point the toes on the lift and reach out away from the body.

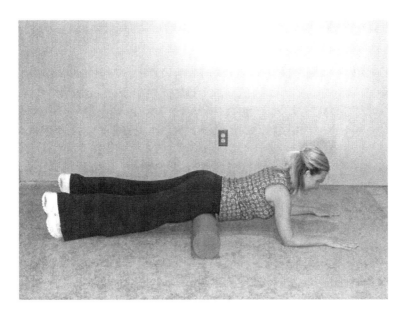

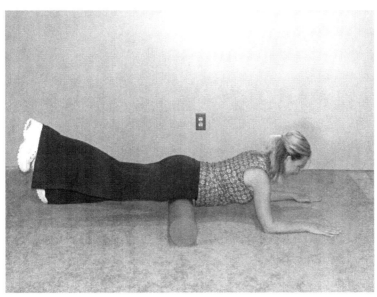

Spinal Balance

Place the roller horizontally on the floor. Kneeling in front of the roller, place your hands shoulder-distance apart on it. Position your knees directly below the hips so that the spine is straight. Exhale and extend a straight right arm and straight left leg until they are parallel to the floor. Inhale and release your arm and leg to the start position. Exhale and extend a straight left arm and straight right leg until they are parallel to the floor. Inhale and release your arm and leg to the start position. Complete the repetitions. For a variation, place the roller underneath the knees (see bottom photo on the next page).

TIPS FROM LISA:

- Tighten the stomach to keep the spine straight.
- Reach out through the fingers and toes to lengthen the spine.

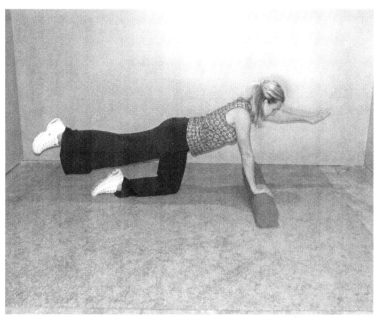

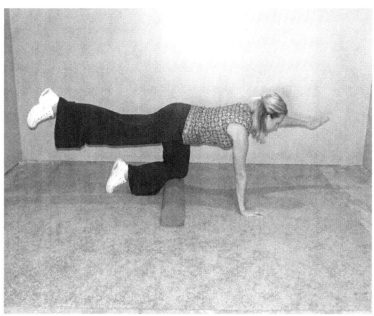

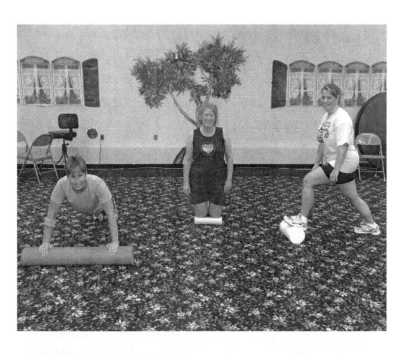

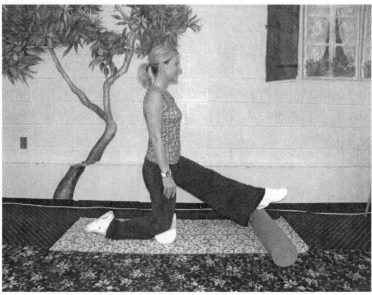

YOGA AND PILATES WITH ROLLERS

How will rollers benefit a yoga workout?

The inherent goal of yoga is to unite the body and the mind. In order to keep the body's alignment in each pose, the mind is passively focused on every small movement. Joint position awareness is crucial for proper alignment and the use of a roller increases this awareness through its unstable surface. Training on this surface activates the mental coordination as well as the physical. The mind needs to be aware of every movement in order to keep the body on the roller.

Strength is also improved through the addition of this prop. Where the muscles previously had only the weight of the body and its various positions to use for strengthening, the muscles now have a new stimulus to adjust to. The core also is activated in every move on the roller, which results in stronger and tighter abdominals.

Rollers also enhance yoga stretching exercises by allowing the body to maneuver into positions that otherwise would not be possible. This improved flexibility carries over into life to improve the quality of daily living, as a supple body is less susceptible to injuries.

On a Roll

While in the exercises, breathe in and out through the nose. Hold each pose for 30-45 seconds or 5-10 breaths. The poses can be repeated as strength and endurance improve. Place the roller on a yoga mat for additional traction.

Downward Facing Dog

Place the roller horizontally on the floor. Begin on all fours with your hands on the roller and your knees on the ground. Press your toes into the floor, straighten your legs and extend your hips toward the ceiling into downward dog. Relax the neck and hold your arms stable with a slight bend in the elbows.

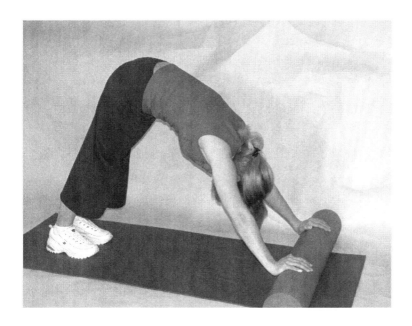

Warrior I

Place the roller horizontally on the floor. Place your left foot onto the roller. Position your right foot at the back of the mat and rest the heel on the mat. Align the arch of your right foot with the heel of the left. Inhale and raise both of your arms overhead, bringing your body upright into Warrior I. As you exhale, bend your left knee to 90 degrees. Hold and repeat on the right leg.

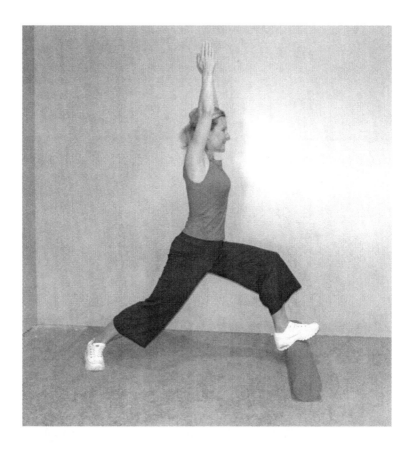

Warrior II

From the Warrior I position, open your hips to the sides and place your arms parallel to the floor with the front arm extended over the front leg. Look toward the front hand. Pull your shoulders away from your ears and bend your front knee to a comfortable position, not exceeding a 90-degree angle. Hold and repeat on the opposite leg.

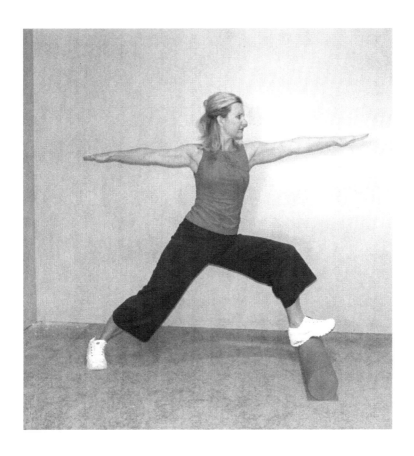

Forward Bend with Calf Stretch

Place the roller horizontally on the floor. Stand with your toes up on the roller and your heels on the floor. Bend forward from your waist and place your hands on the roller. Hold and repeat if needed.

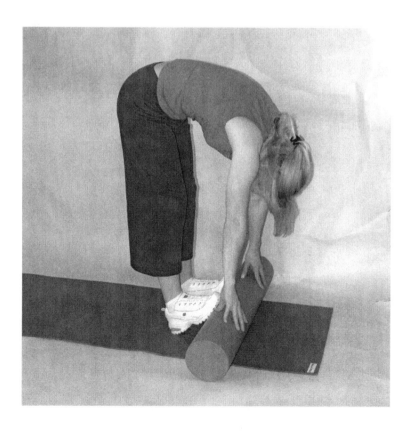

Camel

Kneel on the floor. Place the roller horizontally on the backs of your ankles between the calves and the heels. Inhale, open your chest and place both hands on top of the roller. The closer together the hands are, the more challenging the pose. Look up slightly toward the ceiling, press the hips forward and hold. Release one hand at a time to return to kneeling.

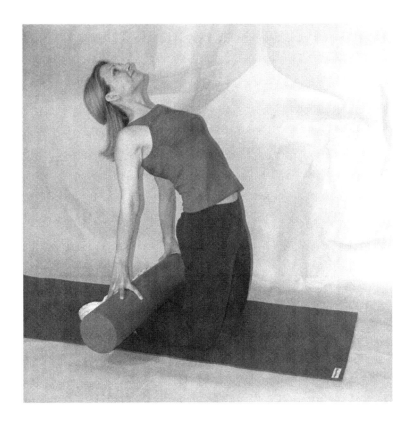

Hero

From the kneeling position in the Camel pose, lower your hips to rest on top of the roller. Adjust your knees to a comfortable position. Close your eyes, relax into the pose and hold.

TIPS FROM LISA:

- Adjust the amount of weight by lifting or lowering the hips.
- Straighten the spine to protect the back.

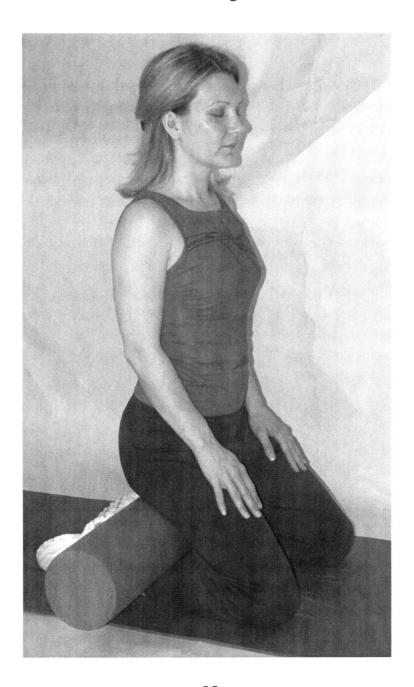

Table Top

Sit on the floor and place the roller horizontally underneath both feet. Leaning back, place your hands behind you, underneath your shoulders, with the fingers facing toward your feet. Bend your knees. Inhale and lift your hips toward the ceiling. Look forward or slightly up. Hold, release and repeat if needed. For a variation, place the roller underneath your hands (see the bottom photo on the next page).

TIPS FROM LISA:

- Widen the distance between the knees if there is any discomfort in the joints.
- Keep the hips pressed up toward the ceiling.

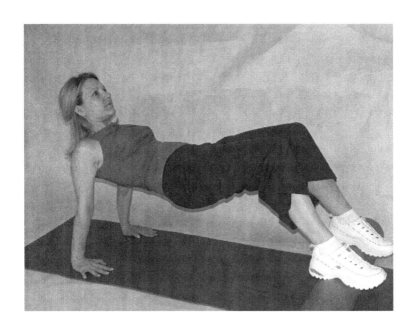

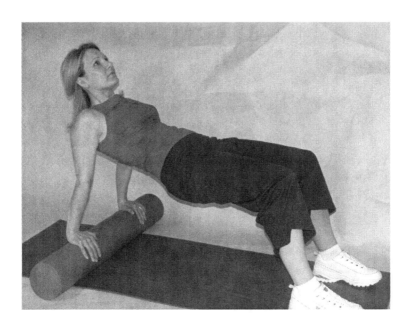

Yoga vs. Pilates

Yoga	Pilates
5,000 years old	60 years old
Mental	Physical
No machines	Machines
Religious-based	Not religious-based
Total body movement	Small focused movements
Total body-based	Core-based
Mind/Body/Spirit	Mind/Body
Inhale and exhale through nose	Inhale through nose, exhale through mouth
Meditation	Perspiration

Similarities

Both increase fitness level, strength, flexibility and health.

Both reduce stress.

Bare feet are used in both mat classes.

Both are helpful in injury recovery.

Both are forms of low impact exercise.

Both use isometric movements.

How will rollers benefit a Pilates workout?

Pilates exercises emphasize breathing, core conditioning and body awareness. The unstable surface of the roller will enhance this core conditioning when the core adjusts to even the smallest roll to keep us centered and balanced.

The improved body awareness acquired with the addition of the roller leads to an active mind/body workout. This concentration allows you to be completely in the moment, freeing the mind of clutter and enabling it to focus on proper breathing.

The rollers will bring added flexibility to Pilates exercise by allowing the body to move through a greater range of motion. The rollers support the tradition of Pilates being a nonimpact exercise. Their lightweight properties are easily transitioned into a workout.

Repeat each exercise 10 times. As strength and control improve, increase the number of sets.

The Roll-up

Place a roller horizontally on the floor. Lie on your back with the roller placed directly below your hips. Straighten your arms above your head and straighten your legs. Inhale and lift your arms toward the ceiling. Exhale and slowly roll forward, lifting your back off the floor. Keep your head in line with your spine. Inhale and fold out over your legs. Exhale and slowly roll back to the start position.

TIPS FROM LISA:

- Point the toes for increased flexibility in the legs.
- Tighten the abdominal muscles for control.

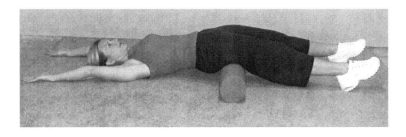

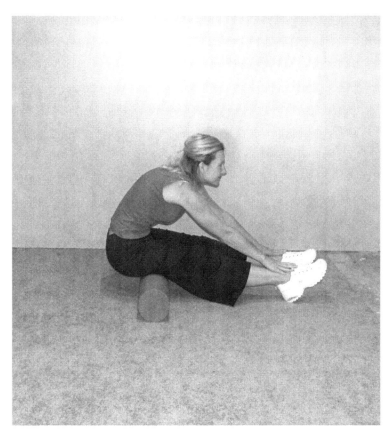

The Hundred

Place a roller horizontally on the floor. Lie on your back with the roller placed directly below the hips. Straighten your legs and point your toes. Place your arms along your sides. Raise your legs, arms and head off the floor. Keeping your palms toward the floor, begin to lift and lower your arms quickly through a 2-3 inch range. Breathe in for five counts and out for five counts. Execute 10 repetitions.

TIPS FROM LISA:

- Beginners should keep the feet on the floor.
- Find a focal point out in the distance for increased balance.

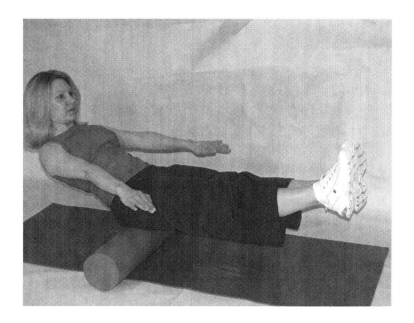

Single Leg Circles

Place a roller horizontally on the floor. Lie on your back with the roller placed directly below the hips. Straighten your legs and point your toes. Place your arms along your sides. Extend your right leg toward the ceiling. Tighten your stomach and begin drawing a small clockwise circle with your toes. Gradually increase the diameter of the circle to as large as your leg will allow. Then reverse the direction and decrease the diameter of the circle to return to the starting position. Repeat on the opposite leg. For a variation, circle both legs at the same time (as shown on the facing page).

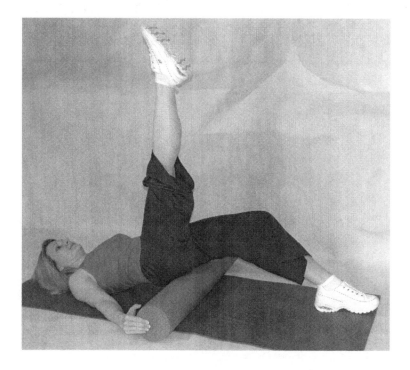

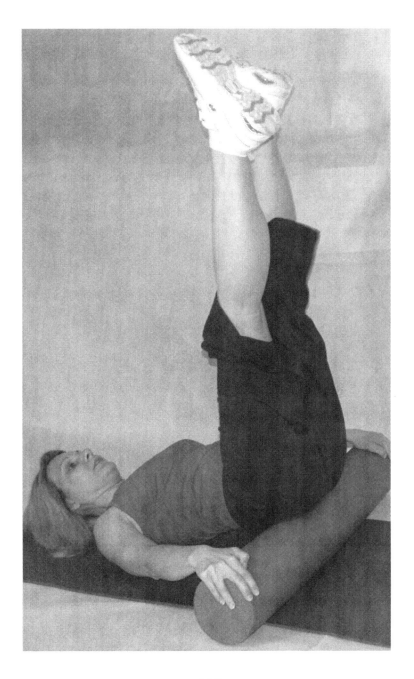

Hip Twist

Place the roller vertically on the floor. Sit straddling the roller with one foot on each side. Hold your arms out to your sides then place your hands on the floor leaning back slightly. As your exhale, tighten your stomach and lift both your legs toward the ceiling with your toes pointed. Inhale and make a circle with both legs. When you reach the top of the circle, exhale and reverse the direction, repeating the circle the opposite way.

TIPS FROM LISA:
- Beginners should lift one leg at a time.
- Keep the focus up toward the lifted feet.

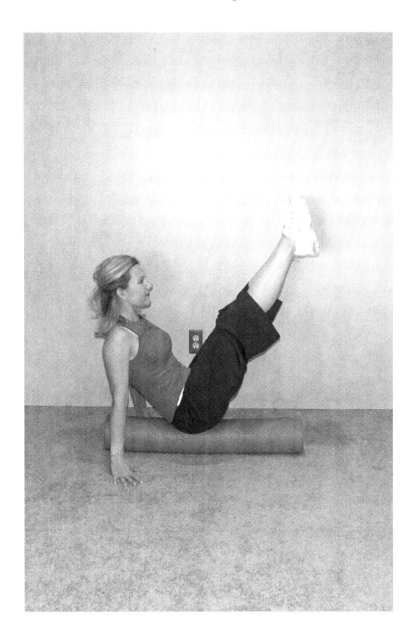

Swan

Place the roller horizontally on the floor. Lie on your stomach with legs straight and tops of the feet on the floor. Straighten your arms in front of the shoulders and place the elbows on the roller. Inhaling, lift the chest off the floor while rolling the roller toward the body and bringing the elbows underneath the shoulders. The wrists will now be on the roller. Exhaling, lower the chest while rolling the roller away from the body until the elbows return to the top of the roller.

TIPS FROM LISA:
- Press the hips into the floor and lift through the lower back.
- Press the tops of the feet into the floor.

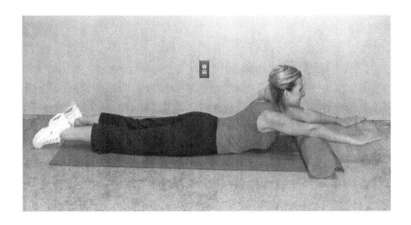

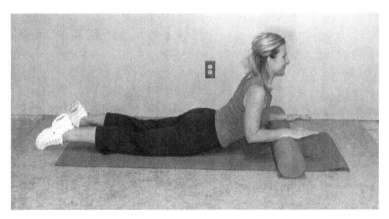

Helicopter

Place the roller horizontally on the floor. Lie on your back with the roller placed across the lower back. Rest your arms along your sides and hold onto the ends of the roller with your hands. Extend both legs toward the ceiling and point your toes. As you inhale, lower your right leg toward the floor and your left leg toward your body. Next bring the right leg out to the right side and the left leg out to the left side. Continue the circular movement to finish with the left leg toward the floor and the right leg toward the body. Exhale and bring both legs straight up over your hips to the start position.

Tips from Lisa:

- Hold on to the roller for stability.
- Tighten the abdominals for control of the legs.

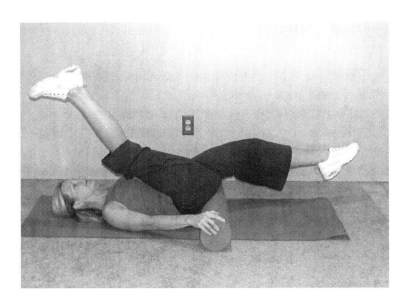

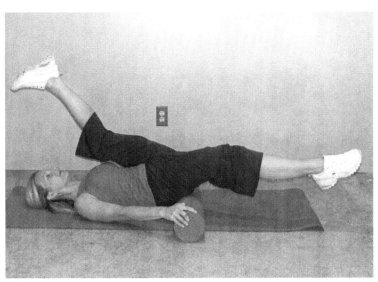

Spine Stretch

   Place the roller horizontally on the floor. Sit on the roller. Straighten your legs and separate them to a comfortable distance. Place your hands on the floor between your legs. Keep your feet flexed and, as you inhale, slowly reach forward between your feet. As you exhale, round your back and return to the start position.

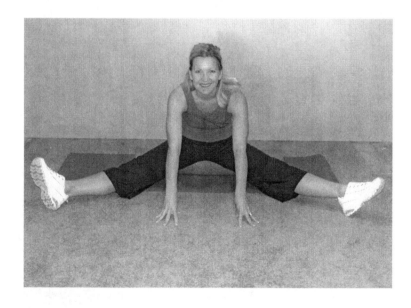

FLEXIBILITY TRAINING

Why is stretching important?

Flexibility is a joint's ability to move through a full range of motion. As with muscular composition, a number of factors can inhibit mobility such as genetics, structure, activity level or injury. Stretching counteracts these limiting factors and helps to correct any muscular imbalances from improper strength training that pull on the bones and shorten muscle fibers. Frequent stretching repairs other imbalances from sports or simple repetitive daily activities.

To receive the most benefits from stretching, daily participation is best. After the muscles are warm, stretching will facilitate muscular relaxation, aid in tissue waste removal, improve circulation and help return muscles to normal resting length.

A low-intensity, long-duration (15-30 second) stretch is favored to alleviate joint stiffness and muscular pain. The stretches are static, meaning without movement. There is no bouncing in a stretch.

Flexibility is specific to each joint, muscle group and individual. The range of motion can also be determined by the time of day. The muscles allow for a greater stretch in the evening after the body has been moving around for hours. Hold each stretch for a 15-30 second count.

Chest Stretch

Standing or seated, hold a roller horizontally behind the body. Place one hand on each end of the roller. Keeping the chest lifted, raise your arms behind the body until a stretch is felt in the chest.

TIPS FROM LISA:
- Open the chest by lifting the rib cage.
- Maintain complete breathing.

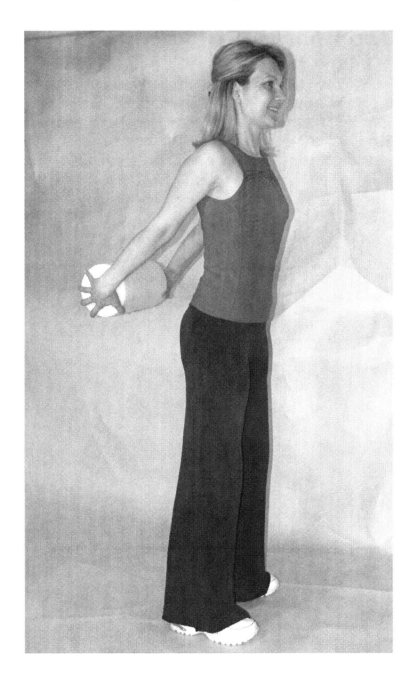

Tricep Stretch

Standing or seated, hold a roller vertically behind the body in the right hand. Place your right hand near your lower back. Reach above your head with your left hand and allow your left hand to drop between your shoulder blades. Adjust the height of the roller so that your left hand rests on an end. Hold, release and repeat on the other arm.

TIPS FROM LISA:
- Place the roller in your bottom hand first.
- Open the chest and lift the rib cage.

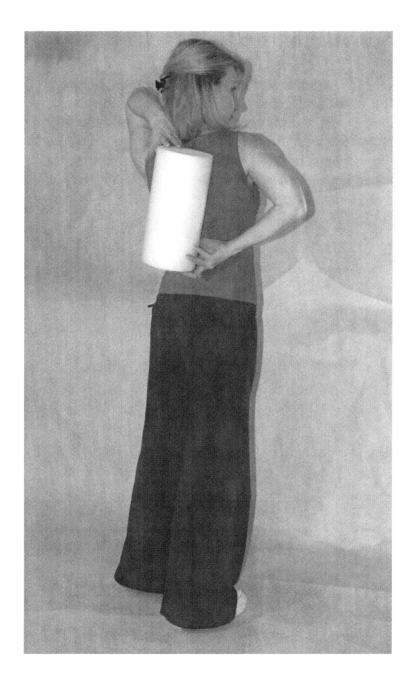

117

Seated Hamstring Stretch

Place a roller horizontally on the floor. Sit on top of the roller and extend your legs straight on the floor. Place your hands on your legs and slowly move your hands toward your feet until a stretch is felt in the backs of your legs. For a variation, sit on the floor and place the roller underneath your ankles (as shown on the bottom photo of the next page).

TIPS FROM LISA:

- Allow the back to round to ease into the stretch.
- Focus on the feet to keep the head aligned.

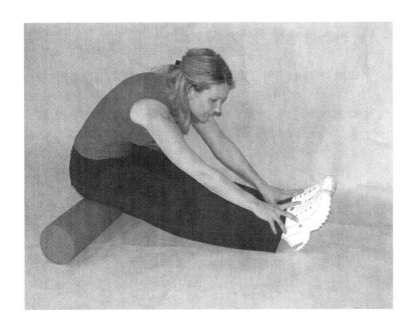

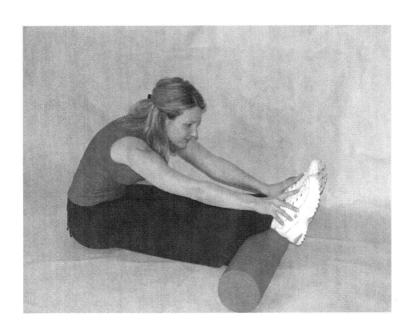

Lying Quadricep Stretch

Place a roller horizontally on the floor. Lie face down on top of the roller, positioning it directly above the hips. Bend the left arm and allow the chin to rest on the back of the left hand. Bend the right leg and reach back with the right hand to grasp the right ankle. Hold, release and repeat on the left leg.

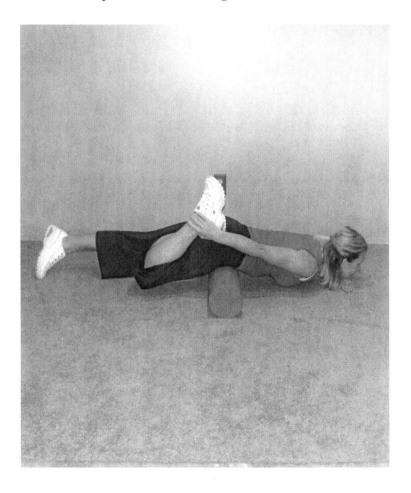

Standing Calf Stretch

Position the roller horizontally against a wall or the back of a chair. Place the arch of your right foot on the side of the roller with your right heel on the floor. Gently bend your right knee and press toward the wall until a stretch is felt in the back of your lower leg. Hold, release and repeat on the left leg.

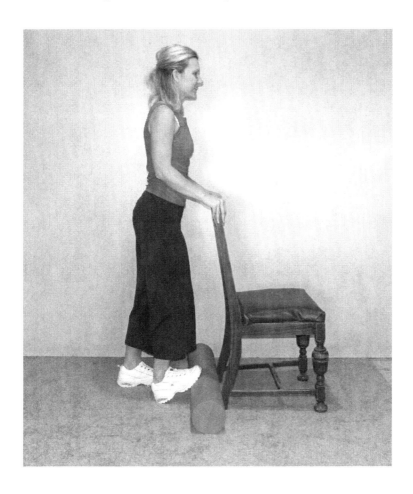

121

Lower Back Stretch

Sit on the floor with your knees bent. Place the roller behind both knees and hold it with your hands. Slowly roll back until you are resting on the floor, and pull the roller toward your chest until a stretch is felt in the lower back.

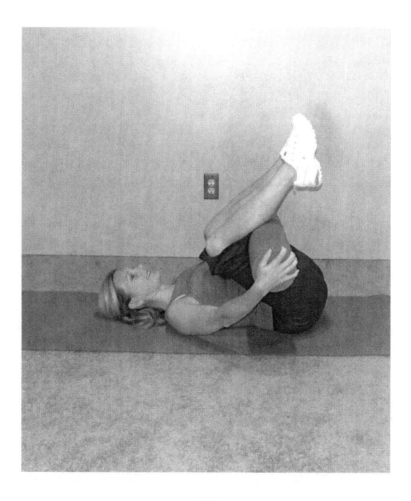

Inner Thigh Stretch

Place the roller horizontally on the floor. Sit on the roller. Bending your knees, bring the soles of your feet together in front of the body and allow your feet to rest on the floor. Hold onto your ankles and bring your feet close to the roller until a stretch is felt in the inner thighs. Press the knees toward the floor.

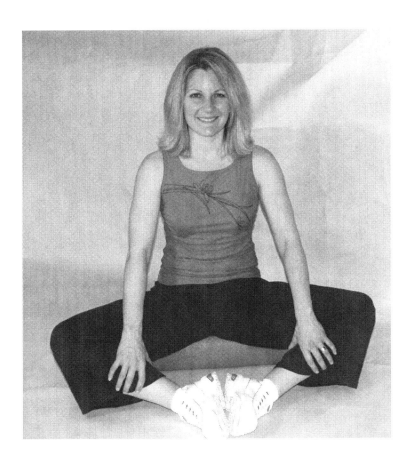

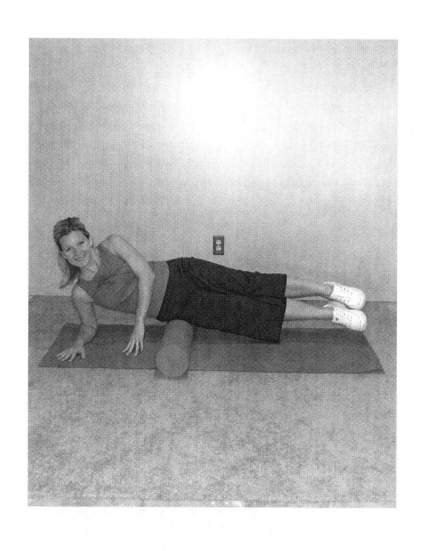

ROLLER MASSAGE

What are the benefits of roller massage?

Roller massage is an effective way to warm up the muscles. It can be used as an aid to prepare cold muscles for deep stretching exercises. The roller's unique design allows it to reach muscles that are difficult to stretch with traditional exercises, such as those along the front of the lower leg.

With regular use of the roller, you will become immediately aware of any muscular tightness that needs to be removed. This early indicator is helpful in avoiding pain and injury.

The roller massage is an opportunity for you to give your body a much-needed reward after a workout. Following the massage, you will feel relaxed and refreshed. The muscles will be lengthened, allowing the bones and joints to return to their proper placement. Also expect to feel anticipation for your next roller massage.

How do I use the roller for a massage?

Roller massage should be performed prior to stretching. The roller should be placed on the muscle tissue, not on the joints or tendons. Begin by placing the roller on the tightest area of the muscle. From there, gradually increase the pressure by relaxing the weight of the body onto the roller. Hold this position until you feel a release in the tightness, but for no longer than one minute.

If an area is sensitive to the touch, avoid roller massage. Also, if the roller does not freely roll up and down the muscle, avoid that area. Follow the directions carefully and if you feel any pain, stop immediately.

Remember to maintain breathing throughout the massage. Close the eyes for more comfort and relaxation.

The Spine

Place a roller vertically on the floor. Sit straddling the roller with one foot on each side. Lie down with the roller along your spine, your knees bent with your feet on the floor and your arms at your sides. Gently roll to the right so that the roller rests on the muscles along the side. Hold for 20-30 seconds or until the muscle releases. Roll back to the center and then gently roll to the left.

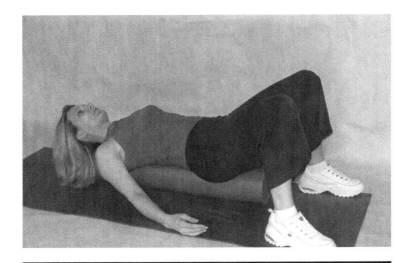

TIPS FROM LISA:
- Widen the distance between the knees for increased stability.
- Center the weight back into the heels, not forward into the toes.

The Back

Place a roller horizontally on the floor. Lie face up with your shoulder blades on top of the roller. Keep your knees bent and your hips lifted off the floor. Straighten your arms overhead. Using your feet in a walking movement, slowly roll the roller toward your hips then return toward the shoulders. Hold on any tight areas for 20-30 seconds.

TIPS FROM LISA:

- Focus on a spot on the ceiling.
- Tighten the abdominal muscles for improved balance.

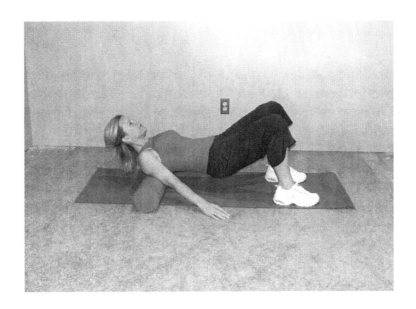

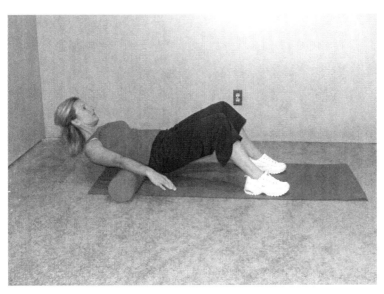

The Lower Back

Place a roller horizontally on the floor. Lie on your right side with the roller between the ribs and the hip. Position your right arm on the floor below your shoulder to support your upper body. Straighten your right leg onto the floor. Keep the left knee bent and place your left foot on the floor behind the right leg for support. Gently lower your left hip toward the roller until you feel the pressure of the roller in the lower back. Do not overstretch this area. Hold for 20-30 seconds and repeat on the left side.

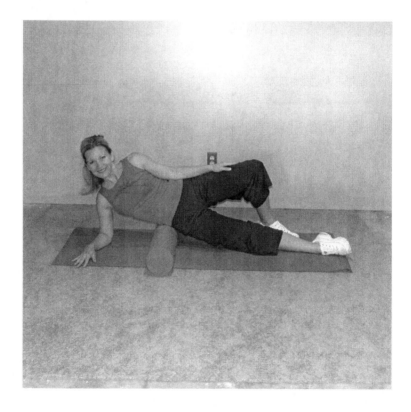

The Chest

Place a roller diagonally on the floor. Lie face down so that the roller rests from the right shoulder toward the left hip. Straighten your legs and rest your elbows on the floor above the roller. Using your arms, roll your body forward and backward over the roller. Hold on any tight areas for 20-30 seconds. Repeat with the roller diagonally placed from the left shoulder toward the right hip.

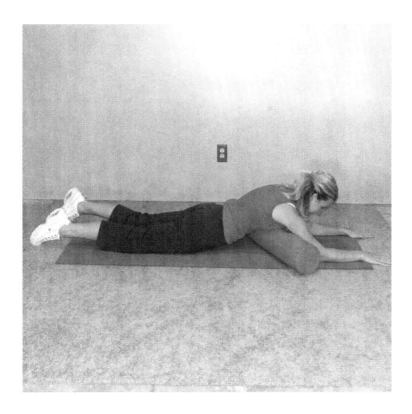

The Gluteus

Place a roller horizontally on the floor. Lie on your right side with the roller placed directly below the hip. Straighten your right leg. Place your right elbow onto the floor. Bend your left leg and place the foot on the floor behind the right leg. Using your left leg, slowly roll the gluteus over the roller. Hold on any tight areas for 20-30 seconds. For a variation, place the left foot in front of the right leg and continue rolling (see the bottom photo on the following page).

TIPS FROM LISA:

- Shoulders and hips should stay in alignment.
- Elbows are placed directly under the shoulders.

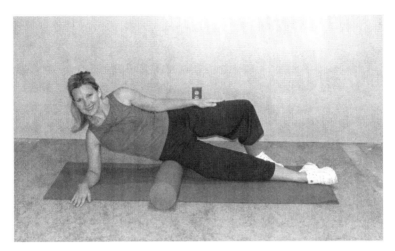

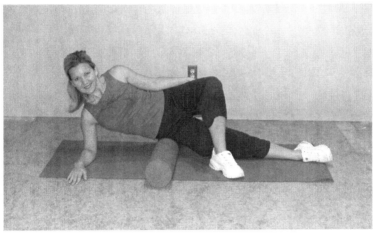

Outer Thigh

Place a roller horizontally on the floor. Lie on your right side with the roller placed at the very top of the leg. Straighten your right leg. Straighten your right arm and place the hand on the floor. Bend your left leg and place the left foot on the floor in front of the right leg. Using the left foot to control the movement, gently roll from the top of the leg toward the knee. Avoid rolling onto the knee. Hold on any tight areas for 20-30 seconds. For a variation, straighten both legs and lift your feet off the floor. Place your right forearm onto the floor for balance (see the bottom photo on the following page).

TIPS FROM LISA:

- Keep the hips stacked one on top of the other, not rolling backward.
- Tighten the abdominal muscles for increased stability.

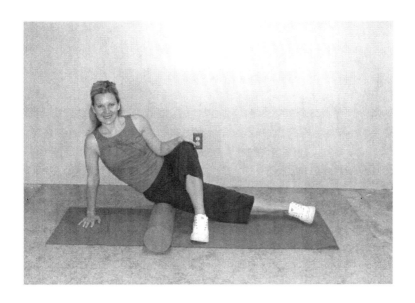

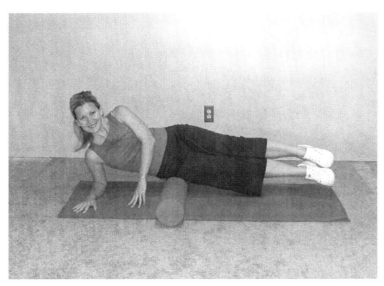

Back of Upper Leg

Place a roller horizontally on the floor. Sit on the roller so it is positioned below the gluteus on the very tops of your legs. Bend your knees slightly and place your heels onto the floor. Place your hands on the floor behind you. Using your hands, gently roll from the gluteus until the roller is right above the back of the knee. Hold any tight areas for 20-30 seconds. For a variation, lift the right leg for more pressure on the left, or the left leg for more pressure on the right (as shown in the bottom photo on the following page).

TIPS FROM LISA:
- Shoulders, elbows and wrists should all be in alignment.
- Point the toes for an increased stretch.

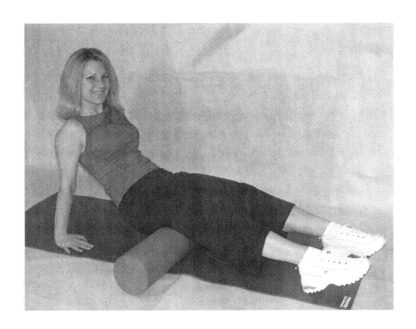

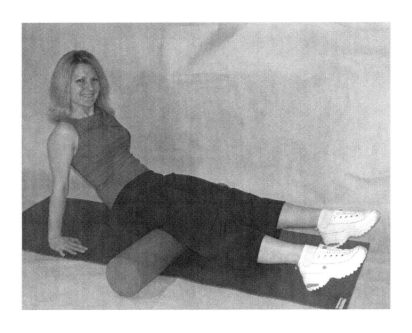

Front of Upper Leg

Place a roller horizontally on the floor. Lie face down with the roller placed at the very tops of your legs. Straighten your legs and rest your toes on the floor. Bend your elbows and rest your forearms on the floor in front of you. Look down as you use your arms to roll from the hips to directly above the knees. Avoid rolling onto the knees. Hold on any tight areas for 20-30 seconds. For a variation, lift the left leg off the roller for more pressure on the right, or lift the right leg for more pressure on the left (see the bottom photo on the following page).

TIPS FROM LISA:
- Look down between the hands.
- Keep the back straight.

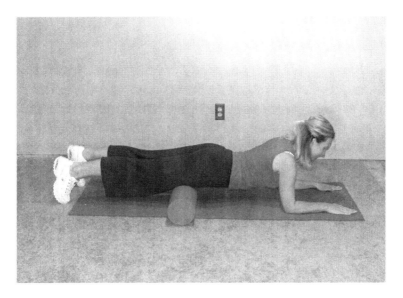

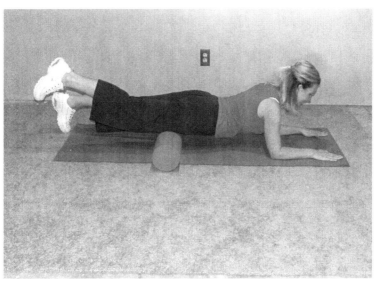

Back of Lower Leg

Place a roller horizontally on the floor. Sit on the floor, straighten your legs and place the roller just below the knees onto the calves. Straighten your arms, place your palms on the floor and lift your hips. Using your hands to move, slowly roll the roller toward the ankles. Hold on any tight areas for 20-30 seconds. For a variation, lift the left leg off the roller for more pressure on the right, or lift the right leg for more pressure on the left (see the bottom photo on the following page).

TIPS FROM LISA:

- Tighten the abdominal muscles to protect the back.
- Shoulders, elbows and wrists should stay in alignment.

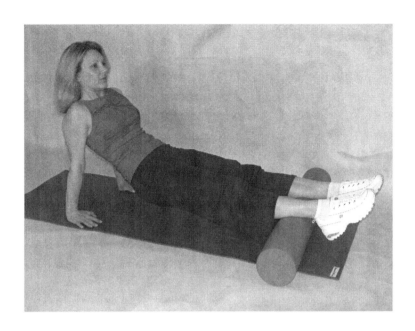

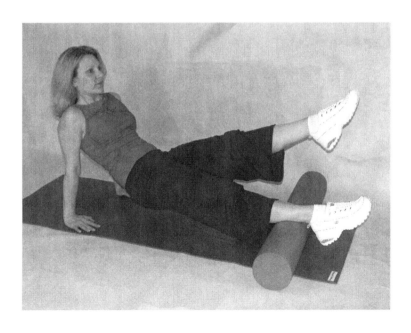

Front of the Lower Leg

Place a roller horizontally on the floor. Kneel on top of the roller and place it directly below your knees. Straighten your arms and place your palms on the floor. Using your hands to guide, gently roll from your knees toward your ankles. Avoid rolling directly on the bones of the shins. Shift your weight so that the muscles make contact with the roller. Hold on any tight areas for 20-30 seconds.

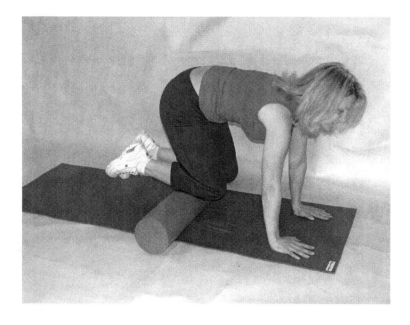

Forearms

Place a roller horizontally on the floor. Lie face down with your legs straight out behind you. Place your arms on the roller directly below the elbows with your palms facing up. Gently roll toward the wrists. Avoid rolling directly on the bones. Turn your palms to the sides to increase the pressure on the muscles. Hold any tight areas for 20-30 seconds.

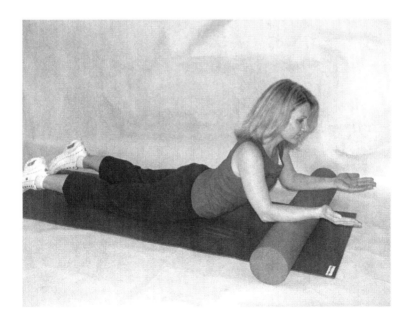

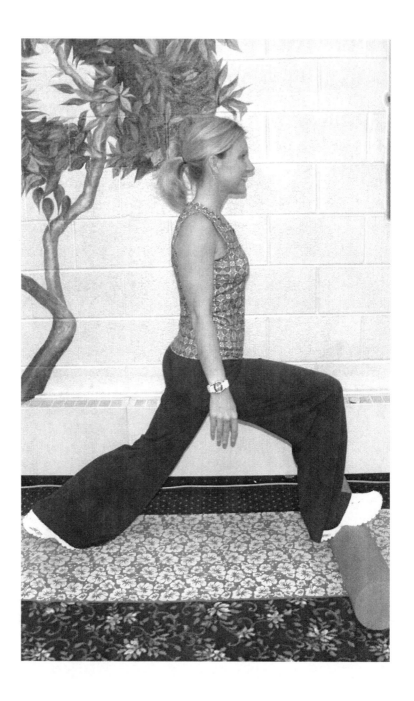

Safety Precautions, Concerns and Modifications

Are there any reasons for not using the roller?

Roller training should be avoided by people with vertigo problems, nausea or light-headedness. Those who have osteoporosis or any weight-bearing restrictions should seek medical advice on roller training. Anyone who has hypermobility, acute fractures or connective tissue disorders such as fibromyalgia or rheumatoid arthritis should avoid roller training. Those undergoing treatment for tumors or taking anticoagulant medication should seek medical advice before roller training.

Roller training can aggravate skin conditions such as acne, contusions, blisters or sensitive skin. Anyone with allergies to polyurethane, vinyl or foam should avoid use of the roller.

What are some modifications for injuries and illnesses?

Those with back injuries should avoid placing the roller directly onto the affected area. During the balance exercises, hold onto a wall or stable chair for additional support. Always keep your spine as straight as possible and tighten the abdominal muscles.

Those with hand or wrist injuries should avoid placing the hands onto the roller.

Those with high blood pressure should avoid squeezing the roller tightly with the hands. Remember to follow the breathing instructions and avoid holding your breath.

Those who are pregnant should check with your doctor before beginning this or any other exercise program.

People with hip, knee or ankle injuries should avoid placing the roller directly onto the affected area. Use caution with balance exercises and hold onto a wall or stable chair for additional support. Check with your doctor before beginning a roller workout.

How can I make the roller workout safe?

Follow the exercise directions and move slowly through the workout. Do not attempt the more challenging variations until you've spent time learning the beginning exercise. Start with a half roller and build up to a full roller.

Always wear shoes and clothes during the workout. Take a rest when you feel you need one. Keep water on hand for hydration and avoid eating for an hour prior to the workout.

Work within your own intensity limitations. One of the greatest benefits of the roller workout is that you control the intensity. Listen to your body and respect how the muscles are responding on a day to day basis. Also work within your range of motion limitations. Flexibility will be different for everyone and different on every day. Pay attention to the muscles and avoid forcing the body into uncomfortable positions.

Follow the guidelines for proper breathing. This will help avoid increasing the blood pressure or becoming light-headed.

Aim for an hour's worth of roller workout three times per week. You can also separate the upper- and lower-body workouts. This would allow you to train on the roller every day, yet still give yourself one day of rest during the week to recover.

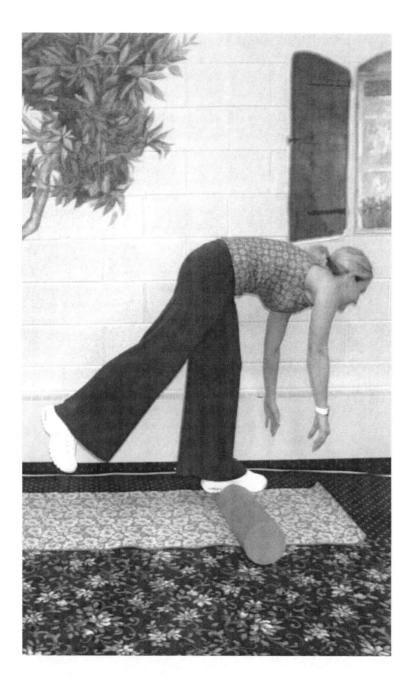

Motivation, Goal Setting and Adherence

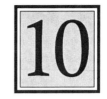

Motivation

Exercise is a very personal subject. Everyone has his or her own reasons for beginning and maintaining an exercise program. At times, even the most dedicated participant needs encouragement to continue. If you find yourself facing an un-motivated moment, here are a few tips that I hope will encourage you:

- There are 3500 calories in one pound. If you burn off 500 calories a day for one week, you'll lose one pound without changing your eating habits.

- Muscle tissue burns calories 24 hours a day, unlike fat, which burns calories only when exercising. The more muscle you have, the more calories you'll burn.

- If you've been active before, it will take approximately one month to make up for a year's worth of inactivity.

- Make the commitment. It takes an average of six weeks to see fitness benefits and 21 days for something to become a habit.

- The way your clothes fit and how you feel are more important than the number on a scale. Throw your scale away if you become discouraged when you look at it.
- Exercise is good for your mind. It alleviates depression, aids in relaxation, lifts self-esteem and helps deal with stress.
- Creating variety in your workouts will help alleviate boredom and keep you seeing the results that you want to see.
- If you're unhappy with your body now, try seeing it as it can become and will be. Visualizing your goal is a wonderful tool for obtaining it.
- Remember—you're a work in progress.
- A year from now, you may wish you had started exercising today.
- Avoid exercise burnout by taking a break to do other things that you enjoy that are unrelated to exercise.
- Keep fit and healthy for your family. They need you.
- Avoid comparing yourself to others. Work out at your own pace and take pride in your accomplishments.
- Get support from family and friends. When you are accountable to someone, you'll be more likely to stick with an exercise program.
- Identify any exercise problems and find solutions to them. Don't let them become excuses.

- The best exercise program is the one that you will do. JUST KEEP MOVING!

Goal Setting

The reason most people never reach their goals is that they don't define them, or ever seriously consider them as believable or achievable. Winners can tell you where they are going, what they plan to do along the way, and who will be sharing the adventure with them.

— Denis Watley

Spend time determining what your goal will be, then fill in the following:

1. State your goal as if it has already occurred. This goal is attainable and measurable. Example: I will spend an hour a day exercising for three months.

2. Write a detailed list of the benefits you will receive from accomplishing your goal. Examples: improved cardiovascular health, weight loss, personal accomplishment, improved self-confidence.

3. Prepare for any obstacles that will hinder reaching your goal. *Examples: Have indoor options available in case of inclement weather. Schedule exercise into the day even when your schedule is hectic.*

4. List people to whom you can be accountable. Have them ask you questions about your

progress. Examples: friends, family, co-workers, other exercisers.

5. Identify your first step in starting this journey. Example: exercising 10 minutes a day for a week.
6. Have fun along the way and release yourself from any setbacks. Start each day with a clean slate.
7. Reward yourself for small accomplishments along the way and save a special reward for the completion of your goal.

This is for your eyes only. Be as specific as you can and be true to yourself and your abilities. This is a tool that can be used again and again to reach numerous goals. The end result is wonderful, but it's the journey along the way that is full of memories!

Adherence

Here are some tips for sticking with your exercise program.

- Always be prepared for exercise by keeping gear and footwear handy.
- Don't expect overnight results or let friend's expectations overwhelm you.
- Have social support from family, friends and co-workers.
- Enhance your exercise enjoyment by varying your program, finding special places to exercise, bringing along favorite music and exercising with a partner.

- Set realistic goals. Think about what is motivating you and whether your program is meeting your needs.
- Make exercise an integral part of your life. It is one of the healthiest choices you can make for YOU!
- Set new goals to prevent boredom.
- Schedule excercise into your day.
- Making the commitment to start exercising is overcoming your greatest hurdle. A year from now, you'll be happy that you started to exercise and stuck with it!

For More Information

To purchase the rollers used in this book, please visit:

Fitness Wholesale
fw@fwonline.com
(800) 537-5512
895-A Hampshire Road, Stow, Ohio 44224
www.fitnesswholesale.com

To purchase the clothing seen in this book, please visit:

Lucy Activewear
customerservice@lucy.com
(877) 999- lucy (5829)
3135 NW Industrial, Portland, OR 97210
www.lucy.com

To reach Lisa Wolfe, please visit:
www.yogaband.com